a woman's guide™ to vitamins and minerals

a woman's guide™ to vitamins and minerals

Sherry Wilson Sultenfuss, M.S., and
Thomas J. Sultenfuss, M.D.

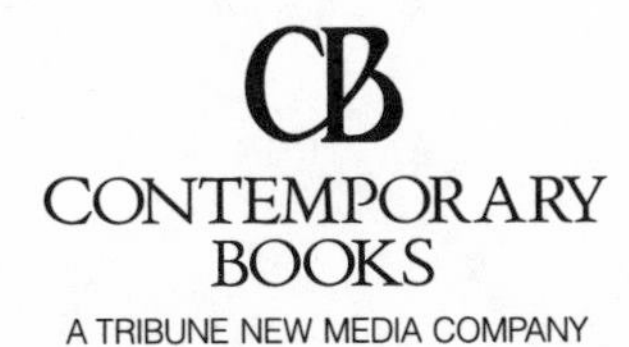

CONTEMPORARY
BOOKS
A TRIBUNE NEW MEDIA COMPANY

Sultenfuss, Sherry Wilson.
A woman's guide to vitamins and minerals / Sherry Wilson Sultenfuss and Thomas J. Sultenfuss.
p. cm.
Includes bibliographical references and index.
ISBN 0-8092-3509-9 (hbk.)
1. Women—Health and hygiene. 2. Dietary supplements. 3. Vitamins in human nutrition. 4. Minerals in human nutrition. I. Sultenfuss, Thomas J. II. Title.
RA778.S926 1995
613'.04244—dc20 94-47604
CIP

This book has been reviewed carefully and every effort has been made to ensure its accuracy. It should, however, be used for informational purposes only. All suggestions and recommendations are intended for educational purposes and made without warranty or guarantee, express or implied, and the author and publisher disclaim all liability in connection with the use of this information. The material presented herein is not a substitute for the advice of a personal health-care professional.

Published by Contemporary Books, Inc.
Two Prudential Plaza, Chicago, Illinois 60601-6790
Manufactured in the United States of America
International Standard Book Number: 0-8092-3509-9
10 9 8 7 6 5 4 3 2 1

This book is dedicated to our mothers, Margaret and Agnes, our daughters, Katherine and Margo, and to all women taking responsibility for their health.

CONTENTS

PREFACE

Throughout my life I have been interested in nutrition, exercise, and basically just staying healthy. I grew up on a farm where we raised our own vegetables for a good part of the year, and my mom saw that the family ate healthy food. Mom made sure we had fresh juice every morning and lots of good, fresh vegetables every day. Looking back, I can see that she gave me a great start, except for the large amounts of meat we ate. Being a child of the sixties, I later had my own garden and haunted the health-food stores. But I was not satisfied with the information I received. I wanted more.

After I had two children in my thirties and gave up any illusions of immortality, I wanted to know what I should do and eat and take as an *adult* woman to improve my chances for a long and healthy life. I could find the answers I wanted neither in the health-food stores nor in the medical or nutritional communities. So I decided to do my own research, and off to the library I went.

There were tons of books on pregnancy. Menopause has

recently been excellently covered by a number of texts, but I was shocked to find so little information on the vitamin and mineral requirements of adult women in general (there is just a tad more for men). The quest for facts began. Pat Jennings, a wonderful and patient medical librarian, ran countless literature searches on health problems common to middle-aged women, and on various vitamins, minerals, and herbs. The information in this book is the result of that compiled research.

After I had finished the first draft, I asked my husband, a board-certified dermatologist, to edit the manuscript for medical accuracy. Although he complained loudly in the beginning about having to put in so many hours of work on top of his practice, by the end he became positively excited about the information. He says his new knowledge in the field has enhanced his medical practice. I am very appreciative of the time and dedication he put into this project.

I am also appreciative for another reason: working on this book has been a joy. I never thought that two independent and headstrong people could work together this closely. I was afraid that our combination of personalities would create an explosion. Instead, with a mutual project and a common goal, we learned a lot about each other and became closer.

—Sherry Wilson Sultenfuss

Acknowledgments

Patricia Jennings, M.S., medical librarian—this book would not have been possible without your time, help, and skill. Thank you so much, Pat!

We would also like to thank the following people for their invaluable help reviewing and editing sections of the book and for the myriad other things needed to make this book a reality: Louis M. Paolillo, M.D., obstetrics and gynecology; Joy Wolff, M.D., obstetrics and gynecology; Nan C. Jensen, R.D., L.D., nutrition; Patrice A. Moreno, M.D., cardiology; Mitchell B. Lowenstein, M.D., rheumatology; Linda Nichols Beyrouti, R.P.T., physical therapy; Anda Norbergs, M.D., oncology; Penny Wise Budoff, M.D., family medicine/gynecology; Katherine O'Hanlan, M.D., obstetrics and gynecology; Marla Russell, R.D., L.D., nutrition; Wulf H. Utian, M.D., Ph.D., obstetrics and gynecology; Michael T. Murray, N.D., naturopathy; Phil Hanna for creative input; William S. Jonassen, Esq., for easing my mind; Alyse Cheney (my agent) for finding me and a way; Walter L. "Skip" Schafer, Jr., just because; Gene Brissie (publishing editor) for sharing a vision.

a woman's guide™ to vitamins and minerals

1

INTRODUCTION

We wrote this book as a review of the scientific literature on vitamins, minerals, and herbs to help the healthy, nonpregnant woman. We hope that this review will arm women with enough information to make intelligent decisions on nutritional choices, including appropriate dosages and the best chemical forms of daily nutritional supplements.

Section I is an overview of vitamins and minerals and how to purchase them. The second section contains information on many of the most common vitamins, minerals, and herbs and how they affect women. Section III has information on bones, cancer, estrogen and hormone replacement therapies, exercise, fish oils, food, the heart, herbs, menopause, PMS, skin, and weight. The fourth section lists the most recent recommended dietary, or daily, allowances (RDAs) of vitamins and minerals, identifies their best chemical form(s) and toxicity levels, and summarizes the recommended ranges of the vitamins and minerals from the reviewed literature. Also included is a summary of nutritional guidelines from the research.

The ultimate goal of nutrition is optimal health. Good nutrition is not a diet that avoids deficiencies but rather one that enhances health. Good nutrition helps the body work more efficiently and improves long-term health. Unfortunately research is quite limited regarding the effects of vitamins, minerals, and herbs on women's health. Many scientific studies are conducted exclusively on men or animals, for therapeutic investigation, or to determine deficiency and toxicity levels rather than to establish levels needed for optimal health. To further complicate matters, evidence is growing that our vitamin requirements change as we age. It has been suggested that the present RDAs be readdressed for the elderly. They appear to be too low for vitamin D, riboflavin, B_6, and B_{12}; they may be too high for vitamin A.[1]

Controlled studies on optimal health are very difficult to design. To find truly reliable data, longitudinal studies over decades need to be conducted. It is extremely difficult to account for all the variables in life that confound this type of study. Therefore, much of the present information on daily intake of vitamins, minerals, and herbs is extrapolated from other studies. For example, high doses of vitamin E have been shown to reduce some of the damage of *atherosclerosis* (hardening and clogging of the arteries). However, it is not known if such high doses of vitamin E are safe to take on a long-term basis or even how high the optimal effective dose is. Information is available on vitamin and mineral dosages that lead to deficiencies and on dosages that are toxic, but there is not much information on dosages for optimal health.

We must all rely on our judgment based on research to choose the best nutritional diet and supplementation program. We should be wary of fads and of companies that make remarkable claims to fix our health problems. We must be careful not to overdose ourselves on any vitamin or mineral. When we take a supplement, balancing the components is imperative. They can interact with one another, and some combinations and dosages may be synergistically beneficial or harmful. There is evidence that taking large doses of one vitamin or mineral will cause a deficiency in another. For example, large doses of zinc will increase the loss of copper and iron.

Fortunately many more research dollars are now being allocated to the study of vitamins, minerals, and herbs. Many of the disputed areas of research will be resolved in the future. Until then, it is up to each of us to make smart choices.

This book is not a medical text; it is a review of some of the scientific literature. No prescriptions are given. The nutritional suggestions in the book are collated from numerous researchers, physicians, and nutritionists. While many of the studies reviewed are controversial and the conclusions may be disputed, the sources of information are mostly from medical and nutritional journals.

I

The Hows and Whys of Vitamin and Mineral Supplements

2

Vitamins and How to Buy Them

Are Supplements Necessary?

Vitamins are organic compounds found in plant and animal food sources; they are necessary *in small amounts* for health and maintenance of body tissues. They must be present in the diet or in supplements since the human body cannot manufacture them. *Hormones* also are needed in small amounts for the same general purposes, but they are manufactured in the body. *Minerals* are naturally occurring, inorganic substances.

An argument has raged for years over the nature and definition of a vitamin. The key to the argument is the phrase *in small amounts*. Recommended vitamin dosages have been defined in the past as the dosages necessary to prevent specific deficiency diseases, such as scurvy, pellagra, beriberi, and rickets. But are these the dosages needed for optimal health? At higher dosages, do vitamins have benefits other than the prevention of deficiency diseases? Recent research has some fascinating if incomplete answers to these questions, as we will see in later chapters.

Vitamins A, E, D, and K are *fat soluble* vitamins and are stored in fatty tissues and in the liver. The other vitamins are *water soluble* and are stored in the body temporarily, for from only a few hours to several days. Quite a bit of controversy exists about taking vitamin and mineral supplements. Some people think that we get all the necessary nutrients from a well-balanced diet; others feel that the U.S. diet in general is nutritionally incomplete. One reason claimed is that the soil that supports both plant and animal life has become somewhat depleted of essential minerals, often due to long-term erosion of farmland. Another reason offered is that modern processing and milling of foods remove much of the vitamin and mineral content. Furthermore the agricultural revolution has increased food production sometimes at the expense of nutritional quality. Grains and fruits are larger and contain more sugar and starch but not proportionately more vitamins and minerals.

Whether a person chooses to take a daily vitamin and mineral supplement or not, it is important to eat a well-balanced, varied diet, drink plenty of fluids, limit calories for a specific body size, get plenty of rest (without stress), and exercise regularly. Writing about the above five requirements is all too easy, yet fitting them into a busy life is so difficult. A vitamin and mineral supplement ideally will act, just as intended, as an aid to us in our present and future health. Vitamins are not a cure-all, nor should they be used as a stimulant to give energy or as a substitute for a well-balanced diet.

The Food and Nutrition Board of the National Research Council of the National Academy of Sciences established *recommended dietary*, or *daily, allowances (RDAs)* as guidelines to ensure that most of a healthy population is meeting its nutritional needs. Remember, however, that the RDAs are designed not for individuals but for populations. Other groups such as the World Health Organization, the Food and Agriculture Organization, and governmental agencies of many individual countries also have nutritional recommendations. These different groups do vary in their guideline estimations and recommendations.[1] However, much of the recent scientific literature suggests that in many cases the RDAs are not adequate for optimal health. The recommendations may simply ward off deficiencies rather than enhance health.

Do Women Need to Take Vitamin and Mineral Supplements?

Our bodies need approximately 40 different nutrients to maintain good health. Traditional medical wisdom once said that all necessary vitamins and minerals can be obtained in a well-balanced diet. But researchers can provide evidence that women need vitamin and mineral supplementation if they are smoking, nursing, dieting, under stress, pregnant, heavy menstrual bleeders, or vegetarians or have gastrointestinal (digestive system) problems.[2] A large-scale nutritional study on both males and females found that girls and women were at the highest risk of low intakes for the 11 minerals analyzed. Calcium, magnesium, iron, zinc, copper, and manganese were low, less than 80 percent of the listed RDAs.[3] In another two-year study, about 70 percent of the women studied consumed less than 70 percent of the RDAs for both zinc and folic acid. Another 30 percent of the women took in less than 70 percent of the RDAs for calcium and iron. And 40 percent of the women had inadequate intake of B_6 and magnesium.[4]

Many vitamin deficiencies may increase the risks for some diseases and speed up the aging process. These adverse effects may be partly due to free-radical reactions. A *free radical* is a highly reactive atom or molecule with an unpaired electron. The unpaired electron can cause damage to fats, structural proteins, enzymes, and informational macromolecules, such as DNA, which composes the genetic material of cells. This free-radical damage can be reduced by antioxidants such as beta-carotene, vitamin C, vitamin E, and selenium. *Antioxidants* are substances that slow damage from *oxidation*, an undesirable chemical change that occurs when oxygen combines with a substance. Rusting and spoilage are examples of damage that can occur.

The *free radical theory* was first introduced in 1954 by Dr. Denham Harman. He proposed that cells have built-in protective enzymes that can either detoxify free radicals or correct the damage done by them. In the process of aging, the enzymes can no longer keep up with the damage being done, and breakdowns in the system occur. This process can be compared to leaving fatty food out on a table overnight. Oxygen reacts with the food and turns it rancid. This is similar to the damage done in the body by free radicals. The free radicals attack the body's cells internally and start deterioration. Antioxidants lessen this free-radical damage.

How to Buy a Vitamin and Mineral Supplement

So many vitamin and mineral supplements flood the market that buying one intelligently seems an overwhelming task. To decide which supplements are needed is difficult enough without being confused by the various labeling formats. It is imperative to read the labels and to understand them.

Understanding Labels

An ingredient listed on the label may be listed plainly, or part of it may be in parentheses. The two listings mean very different things. For example, if the item is zinc picolinate, it can read as "zinc picolinate 50 mg" or "zinc (picolinate) 50 mg." In the first example, 50 milligrams (mg) is the combined weight of the zinc and the picolinate. In the second example, 50 mg refers to the weight of the elemental zinc and does not include the weight of the part in parentheses (picolinate). So if you want to take 50 mg of zinc, pick the second example.

The "Other Ingredients"

Bioavailability of a vitamin or mineral refers to how efficiently it is absorbed by the body. Minerals are usually compounded with other substances that affect bioavailability. This compounding process of binding other substances to the vitamins and minerals is called *chelation*.

Back to the example of zinc picolinate. The zinc is chelated with picolinate to make the zinc easier to absorb (more available). Chelates come in three basic types: inorganic mineral salts, organic mineral chelates, and full-range amino acid chelates. (*Inorganic* means the substance is not related to living matter; *organic* matter contains carbon and generally comes from or relates to living organisms.) The inorganic mineral salts are usually oxides, phosphates, and carbonates. The last contain carbon but are found abundantly in nonliving systems. The organic mineral chelates usually employ fumarates, gluconates, citrates, and different amino acids (building blocks of protein). The full-range amino acid chelates are very complex. This new form supposedly presents minerals in their most bioavailable form.

However, opinions differ as to which process is superior. In some cases, the organic mineral chelates and the full-range amino acid chelates appear more bioavailable. This greater absorption is due to a change in the electrical charge of the chelated minerals. The organic mineral and full-range amino acid chelates are also generally more expensive.[5] Despite the doubts of some that the investment in chelated mineral supplements is worthwhile,[6] other authorities are enthusiastic about their benefits outweighing their costs.[7]

There are many *antagonists*, or substances that inhibit the absorption of a vitamin or mineral. How these substances act depends on the vitamin, mineral, or combination taken and the method by which it is taken. Regardless of the chelate debate mentioned above, having a *balanced* vitamin and mineral supplement is very important. Tissue damage and deficiencies can result from taking the inappropriate dosages or combinations.

Some vitamin and mineral supplements contain other ingredients, including food coloring, preservatives, binders, and fillers. Many of these may cause additional problems such as allergies or other physical reactions. Also, we do not know how these other ingredients may react with the body when taken over a long period of time.[8] The problem of hidden ingredients will be eliminated by new Food and Drug Administration (FDA) regulations mandating the listing of both active and inactive ingredients.

Natural Versus Synthetic

An undying controversy swirls over the supposed advantages of natural over synthetically derived vitamins. Some authorities claim natural vitamins are superior, and others say it really doesn't make any difference. Generally the natural ones are more expensive. We found very little actual scientific research available on this topic, probably due to the rather obvious argument that if two vitamin molecules are identical their origins are irrelevant. An ascorbic acid (vitamin C) molecule has no ancestral memory to tell it whether it came from an orange or a test tube. Vitamin E (tocopherols) from natural sources has generally been regarded as being more potent than synthetic vitamin E, but this is because the synthetic form is sold as a mixture rather than as pure d-alpha tocopherol.

Many natural vitamin preparations also include other ingredients, which (depending on the item) may also be beneficial. For example, rose hips include not only vitamin C but also flavonoids, fructose, malic acid, sucrose, tannins, zinc, and vitamins A_1, B_3, D, and E. Unfortunately, even if the label states that a vitamin is natural, as little as 10 percent of the ingredients are required by law to be of natural origin. The laws governing vitamin labeling will be extensively revised in July 1995.

Expiration Dates and Regulations

Check the expiration date! Vitamin and mineral supplements can lose their potency quickly. Many are sensitive to light, heat, oxygen, and moisture. According to current regulations, only 90 percent of the potency listed on the label has to be present at the time of shipping. Manufacturers are presently required by the government to do very little shelf-life testing, and some manufacturers exercise little laboratory quality control.

When and How to Take Your Supplement

Although following the directions on the label is important, it appears better to take a vitamin and mineral supplement three times a day rather than all at once. The water-soluble vitamins have a greater chance to be absorbed and used if they are taken at intervals throughout the day rather than all together. Time-release vitamins also appear to be of value. They slowly release the ingredients into the body throughout the day.

WEIGHT EQUIVALENCIES

Unit	*Abbreviation*	*Equivalency*
Kilogram	kg	1,000 grams
Gram	g	1,000 milligrams
Milligram	mg	1,000 micrograms
Microgram	mcg	1,000 nanograms
Nanogram	ng	1,000 picograms (pg)

UNITS OF MEASUREMENT OF VITAMINS

Vitamin	*Unit of Measurement*	*Definition*
A	Retinol equivalent (RE)	1 mcg all-trans* retinol 6 mcg all-trans beta-carotene 12 mcg other provitamin A carotenoids
D	International unit (IU)	Equivalent to activity of 0.025 mcg cholecalciferol
E	International unit (IU)	Equivalent to activity of 1 mg of acetate form of dl-alpha tocopherol

*A technical but important term implying that the carbon-carbon bonds are put together in a zig-zag fashion, producing a long, straight molecule.

Checklist for Buying and Taking a Vitamin/Mineral Supplement

1. Know what supplements you want and why you want to take them.
2. Check the ingredients and the presence of parentheses for ingredient amounts.
3. Look out for preservatives, coloring agents, fillers, and binders.
4. Check the expiration date.
5. Take the supplement as directed.
6. Do not take megadoses of vitamins without a doctor's supervision. In vitamin jargon, *megadoses* are amounts many times the general accepted doses, such as 20 grams of vitamin C rather than the RDA of 60 milligrams.

II
The Inside Story on Nutritional Supplements

3

VITAMIN A

PRIMARY FUNCTIONS

Prevents night blindness and other eye disorders
Keeps skin moist and elastic (including the eyes and vagina)
Maintains healthy hair, skin, gums
May reduce risk of breast cancer (large doses of vitamin A as beta-carotene)
Helps alleviate *mastodynia*, or sore breasts (large doses as beta-carotene)
May reduce the risk of lung cancer (large doses as beta-carotene)
Maintains cell structure and integrity[1]
Works as an antioxidant to prevent cell aging and possibly atherosclerosis[2] (large doses as beta-carotene)
Helps prevent infection[3]
Derivatives treat acne, fine skin wrinkling, and the effects of sun damage

Night blindness was recognized as a disease centuries ago by the early Egyptians, but not until this century was the preventative agent found to be a fat-soluble compound present in egg yolks, butter, and fish oil.[4] Today vitamin A is the subject of many different and varied research projects, including exploring its possible value in reducing a woman's risk of breast cancer.

Vitamin A is a fat-soluble vitamin. The term *vitamin A* is used to include *retinol* and a group of chemically similar compounds referred to as "retinoids." They are found in animal products and are toxic at high dosages. Vitamin A as *beta-carotene* is found mostly in fruits and vegetables and is not toxic at any known dose. Beta-carotene is a *provitamin*; it is only turned into retinol as the body requires. Beta-carotene is probably at least as important as retinol in maintaining health.

Some very interesting links have been shown between beta-carotene plasma (blood) levels and the occurrence of cancer.[5] Beta-carotene is known to be a very powerful antioxidant that protects membranes from free-radical damage, while retinol strongly influences *epithelial* tissue (skin, membrane, lining of internal organs) growth.[6] However, beta-carotene, not retinol, may be a protective factor against breast cancer. A New York study, examining 439 postmenopausal (after the final menstrual period) breast cancer patients, found the highest risk in women who had low intakes of beta-carotene. Retinol was not considered a risk factor.[7] On the other side of the world, in Moscow, researchers came to similar conclusions. They found that people who consumed large amounts of animal products were at greater risk for breast cancer. Individuals who had high intakes of fruits and vegetables had a low risk for breast cancer.[8] Again, in Singapore, similar results were found, but only in premenopausal women. This case-controlled study of 200 patients with breast cancer found that the high-risk factor for cancer was a high consumption of red meat. The low-risk factors for cancer were a high consumption of dietary protein from soybean products, high intakes of polyunsaturated fats, and high intake of beta-carotene.[9]

On the other hand, the data regarding retinol and cancers are much less clear. Retinol normalizes the maturation of epithelial tissues such as skin and mucous membranes (moist membranes, such as linings of the mouth and vagina) and therefore is usually thought to have a protective effect against epithelial cancers. However, some studies actually point to a statistical association between high retinol levels and certain cancers, bringing up the possibility that retinol may promote cancer development under some circumstances, especially when coupled with alcohol. Other reasons for the apparent association may be flawed or biased study designs and the fact that liver, the main dietary source of retinol in the United States, is also the most likely to concentrate environmental toxins.[10]

A study examining childhood and adult eating patterns found that the risks of cancer varied depending on age, weight, and diet. Postmenopausal women had a reduced risk of cancer if their diet had high levels of beta-carotene, specifically from carrots. In the same study, an association was found between girls having a heavier weight in childhood and adolescence and a lower risk of premenopausal breast cancer. Yet heavier adult women had increased risk of postmenopausal breast cancer.[11]

Beta-carotene and retinol have also been found useful in treating women with premenopausal mastodynia.[12]

Many studies indicate that low levels of beta-carotene (from fruits and vegetables) increase the risk of lung cancer.[13] Also, smokers who have a diet high in beta-carotene may be protected slightly more from the carcinogenic effects of smoking cigarettes than smokers with low beta-carotene levels.[14] However, the recently released results of the now famous Finnish smokers study published in April 1994 contradict these findings.[15] This randomized, double-blind trial (neither subjects nor evaluators know who has the active or inactive agent until the study is over) followed smokers for five to eight years to see the effects of beta-carotene and vitamin E supplementation. Even the authors of the study were surprised to find that the beta-carotene group actually had a *higher* incidence of lung cancer than the *placebo* group (those who receive an inactive substance for comparison to experimental groups), leading to the uneasy conclusion that beta-carotene may actually be carcinogenic (cancer-causing). No one has a ready explanation for these totally unexpected findings, considering that over 100 previous *epidemiologic studies* (studies of the behavior of diseases in populations) have shown a link between high beta-carotene levels and reduced cancer risks. One of the most recent, also a double-blind, placebo-controlled study, was done in Linxian, China. It showed an overall reduction of 13 percent in cancer mortality.[16]

In another study, involving 1,271 subjects over 65 without cancer, future mortality from cancer appeared to be dependent on the consumption of foods high in beta-carotene. The individuals with low levels had the highest death rate due to cancer.[17]

In light of this conflict, everyone is waiting for the other shoe to drop, since several large trials are currently under way.[18] All this said, however, it appears obvious that nothing will dramatically reduce the risk of lung cancer but to quit smoking.

Topical (applied to the skin) and systemic (administered orally or injected) derivatives of vitamin A (called retinoids) have been used successfully to treat acne and sun-damaged skin. (See Chapter 33 for further information.) Researchers are presently working on other vitamin A derivatives to help heal wounds and treat skin diseases such as psoriasis, actinic keratoses, and leukoplakia. The latter two are precancerous conditions of the skin and mucous membranes.

Food Sources of Beta-Carotene

Green leafy vegetables, carrots, broccoli, tomatoes, sweet potatoes, apricots, watermelons, cantaloupes, and papayas contain beta-carotene. The amount of the vitamin in the fruit or vegetable is dependent on the quality of the soil, amount of rainfall, and amount of sunshine.[19]

Food Sources of Retinol

Retinol is found almost exclusively in animal products such as liver, kidney, milk, and fish. Fish liver oil is very high in retinol.

Recommendations

The recommended daily allowance (RDA) is 800 retinol equivalents (RE), or 4,000 international units (IU) for adult women and pregnant women. The RDA for lactating (nursing) women is 1,300 RE (6,500 IU) for the first six months and 1,200 RE (6,000 IU) from six months on.

One study, conducted on 30 healthy men, examined the beta-carotene in foods and supplements. It found that the plasma levels were higher in the individuals who consumed purified beta-carotene supplements rather than foods high in beta-carotene.[20]

Woman's Guide Suggestion

Supplement with 5,000 IU of vitamin A daily and 3 to 5 milligrams (mg) of beta-carotene daily.

Antagonists

Women who take estrogen (steroid hormones that produce and maintain female characteristics) may have higher need for extra vitamin A. High estrogen intake has been shown to inhibit the absorption of the vitamin.[21] Also, women who take large doses of vitamin E may need larger amounts of vitamin A, since vitamin E inhibits absorption of vitamin A. Vitamin A is sensitive to acid and heat, and it oxidizes quickly on exposure to light and oxygen. Beta-carotene also is sensitive to heat.

Toxicity

Taken for extended periods, 15,000 to 25,000 IU of retinol per day may result in signs of vitamin A overdosage.[22] Beta-carotene, at present, has not been shown to be toxic at any dose.

Warning

Vitamin A as retinol is poisonous in large amounts. Acute poisoning with massive doses can result in nausea, vomiting, headache, dizziness, abdominal pain, and even death. Occurring more commonly are cases of chronic poisoning, resulting in a wide range of symptoms including dry peeling skin, sore mouth, hair loss, brittle nails, dry eyes and blurred vision, decreased appetite, abdominal pain, weight loss, headache, fatigue, cramps, increased thirst, abnormal menses (menstrual periods), arthritis, and liver abnormalities. Patients admitted to psychiatric hospitals repeatedly for depression and schizophrenia have occasionally been shown to be suffering from hypervitaminosis A (toxic effects of overdosage.)[23]

Women who are pregnant or planning to become pregnant should not take over 8,000 IU of vitamin A per day.[24] Birth defects have been associated with high levels of vitamin A intake, so check with a physician. Because of birth defects, oral retinoids for *cystic acne* (a severe, scarring type of acne) are ***absolutely contraindicated*** (considered inadvisable) in pregnant women or in women who may become pregnant during treatment.

4

THE B VITAMINS

PRIMARY FUNCTIONS

Maintain skin, hair, nails, eyes, and mucous membranes
Nerve and brain function and memory
Necessary for liver function
Needed for general metabolism
Maintain muscle tone
Required for blood cell production
Required for antibody production
Needed for production of sex hormones
Lower cholesterol
Increase heat tolerance

The B vitamins, if used as a supplement, should be taken as a group in a B complex. The B vitamins work together, and a balance between them needs to be maintained. Consuming either too little or too much can cause problems. In many cases, a deficiency in one of the B vitamins may signal a deficiency in another. Checking with a physician is advisable if you supplement with one particular B vitamin for a specific problem or deficiency.

There are 11 common B vitamins. They are all water soluble and need to be replaced daily. The B vitamins consist of thiamine, riboflavin, niacin, pantothenic acid, pyridoxine (B_6), folic acid, cyanocobalamin (B_{12}), biotin, para-aminobenzoic acid (PABA), inositol, and choline. Three other compounds are occasionally touted as B vitamins: pangamic acid, orotic acid, and laetrile. They are not commonly used in this country and are not considered essential vitamins.

THIAMINE (B_1)

Thiamine keeps collagen-rich connective tissues and mucous membranes healthy and helps to maintain smooth muscle. (Collagen, the most abundant protein in the body, is the major structural protein providing strength and form to tissues.) Thiamine is known to help in the formation of the blood cells and also is necessary for nervous system function. Low levels of thiamine can cause memory loss and mental deterioration. The classic deficiency disease, seen in people living on polished rice, is called *beriberi.* Two forms occur, with weakness, confusion, and either swelling or wasting, depending on whether the primary tissue damage is heart or nerve tissue. *Wernicke-Korsakoff syndrome*, with nerve damage and memory loss, is seen occasionally in this country in alcoholics.

Food Sources of Thiamine

Whole grains and unmilled rice are high in thiamine, as are beans and seafood.

Recommendations

The recommended daily allowance (RDA) for women aged 25–50 is 1.1 milligrams (mg) and from age 51 up is 1.0 mg. The RDA for pregnant women is 1.5 mg; for lactating women it is 1.6 mg.

Woman's Guide Suggestion

Supplement with 15 mg of thiamine daily.

Antagonists

Dieting and alcohol consumption are main antagonists. Raw fish, coffee, tea, and betel nuts contain enzymes that destroy thiamine. The milling of rice and grains, cooking, and alkaline or acidic pH either inhibit or diminish the available thiamine. Folate (folic acid) deficiency decreases the absorption of thiamine.[1]

Toxicity

Thiamine can be ingested in large quantities without known problems, but large injected doses can rarely cause a reaction resembling ***anaphylactic shock*** (sudden collapse with respiratory distress and circulation failure).[2]

RIBOFLAVIN (B_2)

Riboflavin is necessary for healthy hair, nails, and mucous membranes. It is also important in red blood cell formation, antibody production, and overall growth.

Food Sources of Riboflavin

Many foods contain riboflavin, including meat, eggs, legumes, fish, poultry, green leafy vegetables, and fruits.

Recommendations

The RDA for women between the ages of 25 and 50 is 1.3 mg and for women 51 and older is 1.2 mg. The RDA for pregnant women is 1.6 mg; for lactating women in the first six months it is 1.8 mg, and from six months on it is 1.7 mg.

Woman's Guide Suggestion

Supplement with 15 mg of riboflavin daily.

Antagonists

Sodium bicarbonate, an ingredient used to keep the green color in preserved vegetables, inhibits riboflavin absorption. Riboflavin is sensitive to light and to both acidic and alkaline environments. Also, soaking vegetables in water will leach out riboflavin.

Toxicity

There have been no reports of toxicity from riboflavin.

Warning

Women who exercise excessively or drink alcohol may need extra riboflavin. Women with *hypothyroidism* (low thyroid) are also at risk of having low levels of riboflavin.

NIACIN (B_3)

Niacin is a generic name for a group of compounds that exhibit niacin activity. Nicotinic acid and niacinamide are most commonly used as supplements. Nicotinic acid comes from plants, and niacinamide comes from animal products. It is important to note that nicotinic acid but not niacinamide will raise high-density lipoproteins (*HDLs*). HDLs transport cholesterol from the tissues to the liver, where it can be processed. High HDL levels are considered protective against ***atherosclerosis***, a disease of the arteries. Lesions in the inner walls become thick and hard, and the walls fill with plaque (fat, cholesterol, etc.). As the blood flow is restricted the chance of thrombosis (blood clots) increases.

Nicotinic acid will cause a harmless warm flush that may be disturbing to some women. However, some authors claim that taking an aspirin prior to the niacin reduces flushing. Niacinamide does not evoke a flushing response. Another important chemical, tryptophan, is turned into niacin within the body. ***Tryptophan*** is an amino acid found in both meats and vegetables.

In 1989 a problem appeared in some people taking l-tryptophan supplements, causing damage to nerves, brain, lungs, muscles, and heart. This apparently was traced to a contaminant in the supplements produced by one manufacturer. Despite the fact that the disorder was traced to a contaminant and not to l-tryptophan, the U.S. Food and Drug Administration (FDA) pulled all l-tryptophan supplements off the market because of safety concerns.

Niacin helps in the production of most of the sex hormones. It dilates blood vessels, lowers cholesterol, and aids overall circulation. Supplementation with 3 to 4 grams (g) per day of niacin elevates HDLs.[3] Further research has found that niacin at a dosage of 1 g per day helps reduce the incidence of recurrent ***myocardial infarction*** (the classic heart attack, when the ***myocardium***, or heart muscle, is damaged or destroyed due to restriction or loss of blood supply).[4]

Severe, sustained niacin deficiency results in ***pellagra***, marked by the "three Ds"—diarrhea, dementia (craziness caused by an organic rather than a psychiatric disorder), and dermatitis—and sometimes a fourth D, death. Pellagra used to be seen in the U.S. Southwest among the Native American population, which subsisted almost exclusively on corn, but now is seen mostly in inveterate alcoholics.

Food Sources of Niacin

Niacin is found mostly in meats, fish, and poultry.

Recommendations

The RDA for women ages 25–50 is 15 mg and for women 51 and up is 13 mg. The RDA for pregnant women is 17 mg; for lactating women it is 20 mg. For reducing bad cholesterol in high-cholesterol patients, sustained-release niacin preparations were found to be more effective than the immediate-release type.[5]

Woman's Guide Suggestion

Under the age of 40, supplement with 30 mg of niacin daily, with 100 mg daily after age 40.

Toxicity

Nicotinic acid can cause various problems at levels of 3 to 9 g per day, including pigmentation and dryness of skin and, rarely, liver toxicity and elevated uric acid levels.[6]

Warning

Individuals with ulcers, liver disease, gout, or heart problems should consult a doctor before adding a supplement to the diet. Because of reported liver toxicity, periodic monitoring of liver enzymes may be advisable if you are taking sustained-release niacin.[7] Women who drink alcohol may need extra supplementation. Deficiencies of B_6 and riboflavin will prevent tryptophan from being converted into niacin.

PANTOTHENIC ACID (B_5)

Pantothenic acid has a wide variety of uses. It is important for the production of adrenal gland hormones and supposedly increases overall energy levels; it helps convert food into energy. Found in almost all foods, it is utilized in every tissue of the body. Pantothenic acid is known as the "antistress" vitamin.

Food Sources of Pantothenic Acid

B_5 is found in whole wheat, beans, fresh-water fish, meats, and fresh vegetables.

Recommendations

The RDA given for the safe and adequate intake of B_5 is from 4 to 7 mg.

Woman's Guide Suggestion

Supplement with 25 mg of B_5 daily.

Toxicity

Ten g per day of B_5 have been reported to cause diarrhea and water retention.[8] Other toxic reactions are unknown.

PYRIDOXINE (B_6)

B_6 actually refers to three different compounds: pyridoxine, pyridoxamine, and pyridoxal. B_6 is probably involved in at least 100 different reactions in the body, from the production of the nucleic acids RNA and DNA to relieving water retention. There are conflicting studies on the beneficial effect of high doses of B_6 on premenstrual syndrome (PMS) symptoms.

Food Sources of Pyridoxine

B_6 occurs in brewer's yeast, carrots, spinach, soybeans, eggs, chicken, walnuts, wheat germ, beans, saltwater fish, whole wheat, and fresh vegetables. Pyridoxine is found in plants, whereas pyridoxamine and pyridoxal are found in meats.

Recommendations

The RDA for women aged 15 and up is 1.6 mg per day. The RDA for pregnant women is 2.2 mg per day; for lactating women it is 2.1 mg per day.

Woman's Guide Suggestion

Supplement with 50 mg of B_6 daily.

Antagonists

Pyridoxine is light sensitive, and pyridoxamine and pyridoxal are destroyed by high temperatures. Women who take estrogen or drink alcohol may need to supplement B_6.

Toxicity

Problems are associated with high doses of B_6. In the early 1980s, chronic, large doses of B_6 in the range of 500 mg to 2 g per day were reported to be neurotoxic. Since then, doses averaging 117 mg per day for a six-month period have been blamed for severe motor and sensory *neuropathies* (abnormal conditions in the nervous system).[9]

Warning

Alcohol, certain antituberculosis drugs, and drugs containing estrogen may increase the need for B_6.

FOLIC ACID

Folic acid, or folate, is essential in the production of red blood cells, the production of hormones, and the synthesis of DNA.

Lowered folic acid levels have been reported to increase the risk of colon cancer. A 62 percent lower incidence of cancer was seen in patients with *chronic ulcerative colitis* (an inflammatory disease of the colon) who were given folic acid supplementation.[10]

Low levels of folic acid are associated with a birth defect known as *spina bifida*, in which the neural tube does not close completely during the first weeks of fetal development, resulting in an open spine with varying degrees of paralysis and retardation.[11] The U.S. Public Health Service recommends that women who might become pregnant take .04 mg of folic acid per day to reduce the risk of the disorder. However, a woman who has previously conceived a child with spina bifida should increase her supplemental intake to 4 mg per day if she might become pregnant.[12]

Dysplasia (abnormal cell growth, often seen on Pap smears) of the uterine cervix in women taking oral contraceptives has shown improvement with folic acid supplementation. Apparently, a folic acid metabolic derangement may be wrongly diagnosed as cervical dysplasia or as part of the dysplastic process. The problem has been shown to be arrested or reversed with oral folic acid supplementation.[13] However, a later study by some of the same investigators failed to demonstrate the same effect. Various studies have shown that red blood cell folate level is a good predictor of cervical dysplasia, although it may be protective against ***human papilloma***, or wart, ***virus*** (*HPV*) rather than against dysplasia itself.[14]

Recent research suggests that supplementation with folate may help some memory and affective (emotional) disorders in older people, but so far no controlled studies have been done for confirmation.[15]

Food Sources of Folic Acid

The highest amounts of folate are found in liver and other organ meats, some fruits, legumes, yeast, and fresh greens.

Recommendations

The RDA is 180 micrograms (mcg) for women aged 25 and up; for pregnant women it is 400 mcg. The RDA for lactating women in the first six months is 280 mcg and drops to 260 mcg from six months on.

It has been reported that a daily folate intake of 200–250 mcg meets the needs of nonpregnant women. However, 300 mcg of folate per day allows room for a little extra storage.[16]

Folate deficiency is common in pregnant women in specific populations.[17] Folic acid supplements given before pregnancy have been shown to reduce the incidence of neural tube defects in newborns.[18]

Woman's Guide Suggestion

Supplement with 400 mcg of folic acid daily.

Antagonists

Alcohol interferes with folate utilization. Up to 95 percent of folate can be destroyed by cooking, refining, and canning. Folic acid and some anticonvulsant drugs inhibit each other's absorption. Oral contraceptives increase folate excretion in the urine. This may be responsible for the reduced serum and red cell folate levels seen in oral contraceptive users.[19]

Toxicity

Very high levels of supplemental folic acid (100 times the RDA) may precipitate convulsions in an epileptic patient who is on phenytoin (an anticonvulsant drug) by interfering with absorption of the seizure medicine. No significant problems were seen in a study in which women were given 10 mg of folate daily for four months. However, folic acid supplementation of 400 mcg per day has been shown to interfere with zinc absorption.[20]

Warning

Folic acid can mask a B_{12} deficiency, resulting in brain damage. Check with a physician before increasing folic acid consumption. Women who use oral contraceptives have a higher urinary loss of folate.

CYANOCOBALAMIN (B_{12})

B_{12} is necessary for overall metabolism and nervous system function. It is also essential for the metabolism of folic acid.

B_{12} is needed to make red blood cells and therefore is necessary to prevent ***anemia*** (when an inadequate number or mass of red blood cells results in poor oxygen transport to tissues). Complaints of a B_{12} deficiency include nerve dysfunction, spasticity, confusion, dementia, and visual loss. B_{12} deficiencies occur in strict vegetarians, in older people with loss of stomach acid, and in persons with ***pernicious anemia*** (a previously fatal illness due to an inability to absorb B_{12}). The deficiency can take 3 to 15 years to develop, since the body is so conservative with its stores.

Food Sources of Vitamin B_{12}

B_{12} is not found in vegetables except in some seaweeds and fermented soy products such as tofu. In these exceptions, the B_{12} is actually produced by bacteria rather than being intrinsic in the vegetable sources. It occurs mostly in meats, such as beef and pork. Vegetarians often have a deficiency.

Recommendations

The RDA for females aged 14 and up is 2.0 mcg. The RDA for pregnant women is 2.2 mcg; and for lactating women it is 2.6 mcg.

Woman's Guide Suggestion

Supplement with 50 mcg of B_{12} daily.

Antagonists

Alcohol and medications for gout may interfere with the absorption of B_{12}.

Toxicity

There is no known toxic level.

BIOTIN

Biotin is necessary for the metabolism of carbohydrates, proteins, and fats. It is needed for healthy hair and skin. Some say that it will prevent hair from turning gray, although there is little research to support this.

Food Sources of Biotin

Biotin is found in saltwater fish, cooked egg yolks, soybeans, poultry, milk, whole grains, and yeast.

Recommendations

The RDA for the safe and adequate intake of biotin is 30–100 mcg.

Woman's Guide Suggestion

Supplement with 50 mcg of biotin daily.

Antagonists

Sulfa drugs, antibiotics, and raw egg whites inhibit the absorption of biotin.

Toxicity

There are no known toxic levels.

PARA-AMINOBENZOIC ACID (PABA)

Claims that PABA restores gray hair to its original color are not substantiated. It does aid in the metabolism of proteins and in the production of red blood cells. PABA applied topically acts as a sunscreen. It blocks out the dangerous ultraviolet B rays.

Food Sources of PABA

PABA is found in molasses, whole grains, kidney, and liver.

Recommendations

No RDA is listed for PABA.

Woman's Guide Suggestion

Supplement with 30 mg of PABA daily.

Antagonists

Sulfa drugs, alcohol, and estrogen may inhibit the absorption of PABA and cause a deficiency.

Warning

Allergic rashes to topical PABA sunscreens are relatively common.

INOSITOL

Inositol is essential for healthy hair. It also helps remove fats from the arteries and the liver. It has been noted to be necessary for brain function.

Food Sources of Inositol

Inositol can be found in fruit, meat, milk, and whole grains.

Recommendations

No RDA is listed for inositol.

Woman's Guide Suggestion

Supplement with 80 mg of inositol daily.

Antagonists

Milling removes most of the inositol in grains. Caffeine, alcohol, and estrogen inhibit inositol absorption.

CHOLINE

Choline is necessary for the nervous system and brain function; a deficiency may cause memory problems. Choline is also important for gallbladder and liver function.[21] Large amounts can be supplied as *lecithin* (phosphatidylcholine), a commonly used choline supplement and food additive. Lecithin, polyunsaturated fatty acids, vitamin C, and other B vitamins have been shown to reduce the risk of atherosclerosis. See Chapter 5, "Vitamin C."

Food Sources of Choline

Egg yolks, meat, milk, whole grains, and soybeans are high in choline.

Recommendations

The National Research Council has not determined whether choline is a necessary nutrient. However, the American

Academy of Pediatrics has recommended that 7 mg be contained in 100 calories of baby formula. That is the same percentage found in human breast milk.[22]

Woman's Guide Suggestion

Supplement with 50 mg of choline daily.

Toxicity

Large doses can cause gastrointestinal distress, vomiting, sweating, salivation, and a fishy body odor.[23]

5

Vitamin C

PRIMARY FUNCTIONS

- Necessary for the synthesis of collagen
- Fights infection, reduces inflammation, and heals wounds
- Acts as antioxidant
- May reduce risk of heart disease
- Lowers cholesterol
- May reduce risk of lung, stomach, and esophageal cancers
- Reduces cervical epithelial abnormalities (as reflected by Pap smears)
- Inhibitor of N-nitrosamine (a carcinogen, or cancer-causing agent)
- May reduce the severity of colds

Vitamin C is necessary for the synthesis of *collagen*,[1] a major component of bone, skin, blood vessels, and muscles. A deficiency of vitamin C will inhibit new growth and compromise the health of these tissues. Adequate vitamin C is also critical for healthy gums, and bleeding gums are one of the first signs of a significant vitamin C deficiency. *Ehlers-Danlos syndrome*, a disease of impaired collagen production, has shown marked improvement after prolonged treatment with vitamin C.[2] Also, vitamin C is regularly given to patients with skin ulcers to increase healing and shorten healing time.[3]

Vitamin C helps build the immune system and assists in fighting infection. Suggestions have been made that vitamin C reduces and modulates inflammation because of its antioxidant abilities.[4] Vitamin C may be the most important water-soluble antioxidant for protection against diseases and degenerative processes caused by oxidative stress to the body.[5]

From 1971 to 1974 the *National Health and Nutrition Study* (known as *NHANES I*) sampled 11,348 people between the ages of 25 and 74.[6] The *Epidemiologic Study* (known as *NHEFS*) was a follow-up study on these same people in 1984. During the 10-year period 1,809 deaths occurred. Examination of the causes of death indicated that the people who had low levels of vitamin C had higher mortality rates and more deaths due to heart disease and cancer than did people who supplemented their diets with vitamin C. The amount of vitamin C necessary for the increased health benefits was a dietary consumption of 50 mg a day *plus* daily vitamin C supplementation. Higher mortality was attributed more to low dietary levels of vitamin C than to high dietary levels of cholesterol or fat.[7]

Another study, which researched hundreds of males from different industrialized countries, found that many of the men had low plasma (blood) levels of vitamin C. A correlation between low plasma vitamin C levels and a higher risk of heart disease was found.[8]

Vitamin C has been shown to reduce cholesterol levels in a study of 50 subjects taking 2 g of vitamin C per day for a two-month period. Cholesterol and triglyceride levels decreased significantly, whereas HDLs increased.[9] Other researchers have concluded that in order to reduce atherosclerosis the diet needs to be supplemented not only with vitamin C but also with B_6 in a B complex, polyunsaturated fatty acids, and lecithin.[10] (See "Choline" in Chapter 4.)

Cancer is the second leading cause of death in the United States. Some authorities suspect that a majority of cases may be related to environmental factors. The antioxidant vitamins have been correlated with reduced risks of many cancers, and vitamin C has been associated with reduction in the risk of stomach and esophageal cancers in particular.[11] Among the known cancer-causing factors are *N-nitroso compounds*. This family of compounds is found in cured meats and fish, alcoholic drinks, tobacco, and cigarette smoke and is also produced in the body's gastrointestinal tract. Vitamin C inhibits the formation and absorption of N-nitrosamines.[12]

Low plasma levels of vitamin C in cigarette smokers are suspected to exacerbate smoking-related lung damage, since vitamin C has been shown to neutralize harmful oxidants produced in smokers' lungs.[13] Vitamin C appears to protect against deterioration of pulmonary (lung) function.[14]

Studies of otherwise healthy women with false-positive readings on their *Papanicolaou (Pap) tests* (which examine vaginal and cervical cells to screen for cancer) revealed that a significant number of the women had low plasma levels of vitamin C. The authors of one study suggested a possible relationship between low levels of vitamin C and the possibility of the occurrence of cervical cancer in the future. Further research was suggested.[15]

A few years ago vitamin C was touted as the cure for the common cold. The more ambitious claims did not hold up to later research. However, convincing evidence exists that a higher level of vitamin C (various studies used from 1 to 6 grams per day) will indeed lessen the severity and shorten the length of a cold, even if it does not entirely prevent it.[16]

Vitamin C works synergistically (effects together are greater than the sum of separate effects) with bioflavonoids, which aid in its absorption and are antioxidants themselves. *Bioflavonoids*, also known as vitamin P, consist of hundreds of chemical compounds found in plants. Bioflavonoids, rutin, and hesperidin are relatively common ingredients in vitamin supplements. Bioflavonoids are found in the white part of citrus fruit, in rosehips, apricots, cherries, green peppers, tomatoes, and blackberries.

Food Sources of Vitamin C

Sources include broccoli, green peppers, tomatoes, cabbages, oranges, green leafy vegetables, strawberries, and grapefruit. Small amounts of vitamin C are also found in milk, meats, and cereal.

Recommendations

The RDA for females age 15 years and older is 60 milligrams (mg), 70 mg for pregnant women. The RDA for lactating women in the first six months is 95 mg, 90 mg from six months on. Recommendations by various groups around the world vary from 30 mg per day to 120 mg per day. The late Linus Pauling, a well-known but controversial researcher, has been quoted as recommending 2.3 to 9.5 grams (g) of vitamin C per day.[17]

Woman's Guide Suggestion

Supplement with 500 to 1,500 mg of vitamin C daily (one-third of total taken three times per day). Also supplement with 100 mg of bioflavonoids daily.

Antagonists

Vitamin C is destroyed by heat, light, oxidation on exposure to air, prolonged storage, and alkali. Women who use oral contraceptives, take any form of estrogen, are pregnant or lactating, smoke, drink alcohol, or have undergone surgery may need extra vitamin C in their diets. Corticosteroids, nonsteroidal anti-inflammatory drugs such as ibuprofen, and antibiotics may also deplete vitamin C.[18]

Toxicity

The toxicity levels of vitamin C are unknown. Higher dosages will cause diarrhea.

Warning

High doses can cause false readings on some medical tests such as guaiac tests for blood in the stool and tests for sugar in the urine. Kidney stones and gout have been attributed to a high consumption of vitamin C. However, even at high levels, vitamin C does not cause or worsen kidney stones unless the individual is predisposed to them or already has them. It has been reported that abruptly discontinuing large doses of vitamin C can cause rebound scurvy in mothers and their newborn babies, but these reports are poorly documented.[19] Chewable vitamin C can cause damage to the enamel on teeth. Vitamin C increases the absorption of iron. This may not be a problem in premenopausal years but may cause some problems after menopause. (See Chapter 15.)

6

Vitamin D

PRIMARY FUNCTIONS

Mineralization and calcification of bone
Prevention of rickets in children
Prevention of osteomalacia (bone softening) in adults
Bone and tooth preservation and growth
May lower blood pressure

Vitamin D is both a fat-soluble vitamin *and* a hormone. With help from the sun's rays, it can be produced in the skin from a cholesterol compound; it can also be absorbed from foods in the diet. Vitamin D must be metabolized by the liver and kidneys before it is active.

Vitamin D is partly responsible for bone calcification and mineralization. (A tissue, such as bone, becomes calcified, or hardened, by impregnation of calcium or calcium salts.) Low levels of the vitamin can cause rickets in children and *osteomalacia* in older people. Both conditions are abnormalities of bone mineralization resulting in soft bones.

Bone loss speeds up around the menopause. Sometimes women begin to lose bone density even before they actually stop menstruating. Vitamin D is critical in helping to preserve bones and teeth in perimenopausal women, and supplementation has been shown to retard bone loss during this time. *Perimenopause* is the period of approximately two years before and two years after a woman's final menstrual period; it is a period marked by physical changes noticeable by women.

As women age, vitamin D absorption slows down. This compounds a problem, because the skin no longer synthesizes vitamin D as efficiently and the liver and kidney conversion of vitamin D declines. An intake of 400 to 800 international units (IU) per day will maintain in elderly people the same blood levels of vitamin D that are considered normal in young people.[1] These levels of supplementation are considered safe over long periods.[2]

Bone loss apparently is seasonal, as are vitamin D levels.[3] Most people get sufficient vitamin D from natural sun exposure, adequate sunshine being approximately 15 minutes per day. This is a problem for people who live in cloudy areas or at high latitudes, as demonstrated by the higher rate of osteomalacia in Great Britain than in sunnier locations. There also tends to be more bone loss during cloudy months than during sunny ones. One hypothesis is that decreased vitamin D causes a rise in parathyroid hormone levels during winter, in turn causing an increase in bone turnover. A study of 333 women living in Massachusetts found that women who took more than 220 IU of vitamin D per day maintained a constant parathyroid hormone level throughout the year, rather than having seasonal changes.[4] Women in Canada have been found to have low levels of vitamin D and are advised to supplement their diets.[5]

Low levels of vitamin D and calcium have also been associated with increased blood pressure in older women.[6]

Recently the FDA approved a type of vitamin D cream for the topical treatment of psoriasis.

Food Sources of Vitamin D

Vitamin D is found in fatty saltwater fish, milk products, egg yolks, and liver. There is some concern that the current trends in "eating smart" (i.e., cutting back on fatty, high-cholesterol, high-calorie foods) inadvertently may substantially lower the vitamin D intake in some persons. A theoretical concern also exists about the possibility that the recent widespread use of sunscreens may significantly interfere with vitamin D production in the skin in people with marginal dietary intake of vitamin D.

Recommendations

The RDA for women age 25 and over is 200 IU. The RDA for women who are pregnant or lactating is 400 IU.

Woman's Guide Suggestion

Supplement with 400 IU of vitamin D daily.

Antagonists

Anticonvulsant therapy and some liver and kidney diseases can block the positive effects of vitamin D. Sun-damaged skin and darkly pigmented skin slow down vitamin D synthesis from ultraviolet rays, as do sunscreens.

Toxicity

Vitamin D in amounts of 1,000 to 1,800 IU per day can

cause severe problems, especially in young children. These problems include soft-tissue calcification with heart and kidney damage. On the other hand, an elderly patient with *senile osteoporosis* (bone thinning with easy fractures, characteristic of old age) can often take up to 100,000 IU per day without toxicity.[7]

7

VITAMIN E

PRIMARY FUNCTIONS

Acts as antioxidant
Needed for maintenance of cell membranes
Needed for neurological health
May relieve hot flashes
May relieve mastodynia, or sore breasts
May help fibrocystic breast disease
May reduce incidence of mammary tumors
May relieve PMS symptoms
Works synergistically with selenium
May reduce the risk of lung cancer
May reduce the risk of heart disease

Vitamin E, a fat-soluble vitamin, is the generic name for a technical group of eight compounds: four tocopherols—alpha, beta, gamma, and delta—and four tocotrienols. Alpha tocopherol is the most active form of vitamin E.

Vitamin E, commonly known as an antioxidant, protects polyunsaturated fats from spoiling or oxidizing. It does this effectively in cell membranes and is one of the major agents that keep cell membranes healthy. Evidence also exists that vitamin E has an important role in maintaining neurological health. Some researchers recommend that individuals who have fat ***malabsorption*** (faulty absorption of nutrients) problems or vitamin E deficiencies supplement their diets with vitamin E in order to avoid neurological abnormalities.[1]

Many individuals have claimed that vitamin E relieves the *hot flashes* (transient flushing that causes a hot sensation and sweating) associated with menopause. This has not been successfully documented in the scientific medical research, yet many women affirm its efficacy after supplementing their diets with it. Vitamin E is reported to limit the excessive menopausal production of follicle-stimulating and luteinizing hormones (*FSH* and *LH*, respectively).[2] Based on anecdotal information, one author suggested that vitamin E in the recommended doses may work and will not cause harm.[3] Perry and O'Hanlan state in *Natural Menopause* that nutritionists' recommendations of 100 milligrams (mg) of vitamin E, 500 mg of vitamin C, and a B-complex vitamin, with or without 25 micrograms (mcg) of selenium, may provide relief.[4] Ruth Jacobowitz, the author of *150 Most-Asked Questions About Menopause*, states that she personally took 400 mg of vitamin E twice daily, with relief of her symptoms.[5]

Breast soreness, or mastodynia, is a complaint of many women. It can be attributed to a number of different causes, most not serious. However, in some cases mastodynia may be a symptom of more dire problems such as breast cancer. In *Menopause and the Years Ahead*, the authors suggested that when mastodynia results from estrogen or hormone replacement therapy (*ERT/HRT*), women should try vitamin E along with ibuprofen and eliminate all caffeine, *for a week or so only*, to see if the symptoms subside.[6]

Fibrocystic breast disease increases with premenopausal

(years of regular menstrual cycles) age and decreases after menopause. It is aggravated by high levels of estrogen and low levels of progesterone. The symptoms of the disease include breast tenderness, lumps, and cysts. It has been suggested that this disease increases a woman's risk of future breast cancer. Fibrocystic breast disease has been treated with estrogen and progestins or with progestins alone to counter the estrogens. These treatments have also been used in conjunction with vitamin E supplementation. In very mild cases of the disorder, vitamin E alone has been shown to alleviate some of the problems.[7] However, researchers in several double-blind studies concluded that treating fibrocystic breast disease with vitamin E was without benefit.[8]

One review of the literature proposed that supplementation of vitamin E at higher levels than the recommended dietary allowances may reduce the future risk of breast cancer. It noted that vitamin E helped reduce the incidence of mammary (breast) tumors. Whether vitamin E works as a cellular antioxidant, as an agent that improves DNA replication, or as both was unknown, and the authors suggested that large-scale research be conducted.[9]

Another group came to a different conclusion when they examined 120 women with breast cancer and compared them with 109 women in a control group. They found higher serum levels of vitamin E and a reduced level of lipid peroxidation (a type of oxidation of fats) in the breast cancer population. (Lipid peroxidation is low in rapidly proliferating tissues such as cancers.) Vitamin E is a suspected factor in reducing peroxidation levels. This study concluded that high levels of vitamin E are associated with an *increased* risk of premenopausal breast cancer but that the high vitamin E levels may be the result rather than the cause of the cancers or may be coincidental.[10]

A randomized double-blind study on 41 women with

premenstrual syndrome (PMS) found that treating the women with 400 IU of alpha tocopherol daily reduced their symptoms. The women found improvement in specific affective (emotional) and physical complaints.[11]

Selenium and vitamin E have a synergistic relationship. Selenium is needed for the functioning of the antioxidant enzyme glutathione peroxidase, which also protects membrane lipids, and the two need each other to work properly in the body. Presently there is a concern, because of poorer soil conditions, that our diets may be deficient in selenium (see Chapter 21).[12] A double-blind study was recently completed in a mineral- and vitamin-deficient area of China. Subjects supplemented with a combination of vitamin E, selenium, and beta-carotene showed a reduction of 13 percent in cancer deaths.[13]

Research was conducted on 99 people who had lung cancer and 196 normal controls in Washington County, Maryland. The researchers studied the relationships between serum beta-carotene, retinol, vitamin E, and the risk of lung cancer. The results of the study indicated that low serum levels of vitamin E were associated with increased risk of all types of lung cancer and low levels of beta-carotene were associated with increased risk of squamous-cell carcinoma of the lung specifically.[14]

Vitamin E supplementation may increase the rate of muscle rebuilding after exercise, especially in older individuals.[15] Evidence also exists that vitamin E may be helpful during exercise in high altitudes.[16] (See Chapter 26.)

A heart disease study of adherence patterns of blood platelets in healthy men and women found that platelets preferred to adhere to places that had been previously occupied by blood clots. In addition, a remarkable decrease was observed in platelet adherence after vitamin E supplementation. Vitamin E was given as d-alpha tocopherol over a four-week period: 200 IU were given for two weeks, and 400 IU were given the second two weeks. The average decrease in adhesion after two weeks was 75 percent and after four weeks was 82 percent.[17] This may protect against heart disease by discouraging blood clots.

A *blood clot*, or *thrombus*, is a thickened, jellylike mass formed from platelets and other factors in the blood. Normally this is good; clot formation is necessary to stop bleeding after injury. However, people who have atherosclerosis have an exaggerated tendency to form clots in inappropriate places, causing a stroke or a heart attack.

A *stroke* is sudden impairment of brain function caused by either hemorrhage or loss of blood supply to brain tissues. The victim may suffer loss of speech, hearing, memory, vision, or mobility—or may die. In a *heart attack*, the interruption of blood flow caused by the clot leads to damaged or destroyed heart muscle tissue.

Food Sources of Vitamin E

Sources include wheat germ oil, corn oil, safflower oil, soybean oil, wheat germ, mangos, lettuce, green peas, brown rice, egg yolks, liver, nuts, vegetables, cereal grains, sesame seeds, haddock, mackerel, and herring.

The above list, although technically accurate, may not be useful in a practical sense. This is because the necessary daily amount of vitamin E is dependent on the amount of polyunsaturated fatty acids (PUFAs) consumed in the diet. Vitamin E protects PUFAs from peroxidation. So, as the levels of PUFAs increase, so do the necessary levels of vitamin E. PUFAs also slow the absorption of vitamin E.[18] High levels can actually cause a vitamin E deficiency if the diet is marginal in vitamin E. For example, a walnut is high in vitamin E and very high in PUFAs; however, protecting the large amount of PUFAs in walnuts from peroxidation requires more vitamin E than walnuts contain. Wheat germ oil is an excellent source of vitamin E, containing 215 mg per 100 g of oil and needing only 41 mg for oxidative protection. Corn oil is a net wash, needing all of its vitamin E for its own oxidative protection. And safflower oil, widely touted as a vitamin E source, actually uses up 11 mg more of vitamin E than 100 grams of oil contain. This is why people who eat large amounts of polyunsaturated fats need to increase their vitamin E intake.

Large amounts of fish liver oils (commonly used as a vitamin A supplement) also increase the need for vitamin E.

Recommendations

The RDA for adult women 25 and above is 8 mg. The recommended level for pregnant women is 10 mg. The RDA for lactating women in months one through six is 12 mg and after six months is 11 mg. An intake of 200–800 mg per day, which is 20 to 80 times the suggested levels, has been considered safe.[19]

Woman's Guide Suggestion

Supplement with 400 to 800 mg of vitamin E daily.

Antagonists

Vitamin E is quite unstable. Both cooking and storage reduce availability of the vitamin. Estrogen and high levels of iron may interfere with vitamin E absorption. Therefore, inorganic iron or birth control pills should be taken separately from vitamin E.[20]

Toxicity

According to one review, a person would have to take up to 3,200 IU per day before any consistent side effects are seen.[21]

Warning

Vitamin E can produce coagulation problems in the presence of a vitamin K deficiency.[22] Large doses of E may increase the need for vitamin K and result in bleeding problems in persons taking blood thinners.[23]

8

Vitamin K

PRIMARY FUNCTIONS

Active blood clotting agent
Growth of bones

Vitamin K is needed for normal blood clotting. In fact, blood thinners such as Coumadin work by inhibiting the action of vitamin K. Signs of deficiency are easy bruising, slow clotting, and bleeding gums. However, except in cases of severe intestinal malabsorption, kidney failure, or antibiotic therapy in debilitated patients, vitamin K–related bleeding problems are rare in adults. The amount of vitamin K contained in the diet and synthesized in the intestines is otherwise sufficient to prevent bleeding abnormalities.

Actions of vitamin K concerning bone maintenance are probably more germane to the concerns of healthy adult women. Research on vitamin K's role in bone formation has been ongoing, if not continuous, over the past 20 years. A few studies have shown that supplementation with vitamin K reduces calcium loss in postmenopausal women.[1] A 1984 study was done on osteoporotic patients with either spinal crush fractures or femoral neck fractures. It determined that the circulating vitamin K levels were as much as one-third lower than in individuals without osteoporosis. A 1991 study suggested that serum levels of vitamin K may be useful as a tool to predict osteoporosis.[2] More long-term research is needed to further elucidate the role of vitamin K in bone growth and the necessary dietary requirements for humans.[3]

K_1, known as *phylloquinone*, is found in plants and must be ingested. K_2, known as *menaquinone*, is produced in the gut by intestinal bacteria; it is also found in some animal tissues. Vitamin K_3, known as *menadione*, is the synthetic form that can be converted by the liver to menaquinone. Vitamin K_2 allegedly may be more biologically active than K_1.[4] Many of the K vitamins presently sold on the market are in the form of K_1.

Food Sources of Vitamin K

Vitamin K is found in some green leafy vegetables, broccoli, cauliflower, spinach, brussels sprouts, soybeans, coffee, green tea, butter, liver, and bacon.

Recommendations

The National Academy of Sciences first gave a recommendation for a dietary allowance of vitamin K in 1989. The RDA for women is 65 micrograms (mcg). No special allowance was made for pregnant or lactating women. *Most multivitamins do not contain vitamin K.*

Yogurt and kefir (with lactobacilli) keep the bacterial levels in the intestines high, resulting in adequate vitamin K synthesis.[5]

Woman's Guide Suggestion

Supplement with 10 mcg of vitamin K daily.

Antagonists

Androgens (steroid hormones that produce and maintain masculine characteristics) enhance a deficiency of vitamin K; estrogen acts as a protector.[6] Absorption is inhibited by large doses of vitamin E, mineral oil, laxatives, and prolonged intravenous feeding. When given to pregnant mothers, anticonvulsants can block vitamin K and cause serious *hypoprothombinemia* (a blood clotting factor deficiency) in newborns. Antibiotic therapy or intestinal disorders that cause problems with fat absorption can antagonize the absorption of vitamin K. Vitamin K deficiencies are not very common in adults, yet are common in newborn children delivered at home. (By law in the United States, all hospital-born babies receive a vitamin K shot that eliminates the problem.) Vitamin K does not pass through the placenta very well, and babies' intestines are sterile at birth.

Toxicity

Toxic manifestations of vitamin K are unknown except when given as menadione in massive doses to newborns.[7]

Warning

Do not take vitamin K while taking a blood thinner (e.g., Coumadin) without a physician's approval.

9

BORON

PRIMARY FUNCTIONS

Healthy bones
Increases absorption of calcium, magnesium, and phosphorus

Boron plays a possible role in bone formation, and low boron consumption may be one factor in the development of osteoporosis. Boron is thought to be involved in parathyroid metabolism and thus influential in the metabolism of calcium, magnesium, vitamin D, and phosphorus.[1] Supplementation daily with 3 milligrams (mg) of boron markedly reduces the urinary loss of calcium and magnesium in postmenopausal women with boron-deficient diets. These changes are consistent with conservation of bone mass and resistance to osteoporosis. The supplementation also increases levels of serum estradiol (naturally occurring estrogen) and testosterone (major male hormone). A well-balanced diet high in fruits and vegetables should be able to supply 1.5 to 3 mg of boron per day.[2]

Food Sources of Boron

Sources include green leafy vegetables, grains, grapes, raisins, apples, nuts, wine, cider, and beer.

Recommendations

No RDA has been designated.

Woman's Guide Suggestion

Supplement with 3 mg of boron daily.

Toxicity

Environmental poisoning involving boric acid and borates has been reported.

10
Calcium

PRIMARY FUNCTIONS

Builds bones and teeth
Needed for proper heart rhythms
Needed to conduct nerve impulses
Needed for relaxation and contraction of muscle
May reduce risk of colon cancer
May lower blood pressure

Calcium is needed for the growth and health of bones and teeth. In fact, 99 percent of the body's calcium is stored in those tissues. Calcium stores are increased in the body until approximately age 35. The stores are similar to a reservoir, the body filling the calcium reservoir for the first part of life and draining it in the second half. If there has been good nutrition and an adequate supply of calcium, the calcium reservoir should be large enough to last throughout life. Unfortunately, at the present time, no proven way has been found of catching up later in life if the reservoir runs low. It is critical, therefore, in the younger years, to consume a healthy diet high in calcium[1] and to maintain a moderate level of exercise to ensure good bone density.

Babies, young children, and adolescents need a lot of calcium; the major growth of bones takes place in the early years. These bones must last all of us a lifetime. Until about age 60 the body absorbs about 30 percent of the dietary calcium consumed. After that the absorption declines. During pregnancy women use an additional 400 mg of calcium a day and when lactating an additional 300 mg per day.[2] The bad news is that the daily calcium intake for the average woman in the United States is generally less than half the recommended daily allowance (RDA) of 800 mg.[3] Many authorities believe the RDA to be inadequate, citing the relative safety of higher levels of calcium intake, the devastating consequences of osteoporosis, and the fact that modern hunter-gatherers (who live like our ancestors did and have no osteoporosis) have dietary calcium intakes of 1,900 to 2,500 mg per day.[4]

A few studies tried to determine if there are significant differences between the bone densities of vegetarian and omnivorous (eating both plants and animals) women. Results varied. In some studies, no significant differences between the groups were found.[5] Other studies found that vegetarians had greater bone density both before and after menopause.[6] It is known that red meat inhibits the absorption of calcium.

Many studies have been conducted to discover which minerals and vitamins are associated with high bone density. Zinc, iron, and magnesium appear to be indicators of high bone density in specific bone sites.[7] A study from North Dakota found that people in high-fluoride areas had a lower incidence of osteoporosis and higher bone mineral density than those in low-fluoride areas.[8] This finding was supported by another study that compared two Finnish towns: women in the town having fluoridated water had fewer bone fractures than the women in the town without fluoridation.[9] In yet another study, groups of people who had been supplemented with a fluoride/calcium/vitamin D combination had the least number of fractures when they were compared with control groups.[10] Women with osteoporosis have been shown to be well below the RDAs in sodium, calcium, cholesterol, magnesium, fluoride, zinc, and folic acid. They also tend to have a very low caloric intake.[11] As might be expected, women who have or have had *anorexia nervosa* (an eating disorder usually involving girls and women) have a significantly lower bone density than do women who eat normally. Victims become obsessed with their weight and develop symptoms such as a distorted body image, self-starvation, intentional vomiting, and the abuse of laxatives. The low intake of nutrients along with the other typical behavior of the eating disorder causes accelerated bone loss.[12] It has been suggested that the quality of the total diet rather than solely the amount of calcium prevents bone loss.[13]

Calcium and vitamin D have been associated with a lower risk of colon cancer.[14] A 19-year study that examined 1,954 men found the highest risk of colon and rectal cancer in the group of men that had the lowest intakes of both vitamin D and calcium. The risk was reduced in each of the other three groups with higher intakes of the nutrients.[15]

Calcium, along with vitamin D, appears to lower blood pressure. One study that examined 222 women ages 55–80 and 86 women ages 20–35 found that the women who had less than the RDA in both calcium and vitamin D had significantly higher systolic blood pressure (measure of the highest blood pressure, which occurs during contraction of the lower heart chambers, or ventricles) than women who met the RDA in one of the nutrients.[16]

Presently many women are supplementing their diets with

calcium. The results of some studies indicate that if a person has a calcium deficiency and takes a calcium supplement, the bone mineral density is improved slightly. However, in those who do not have a calcium deficiency, calcium supplementation may not prevent bone loss due to menopause and aging.[17] In contrast, a recent study that compared postmenopausal women over a two-year period found that women who were supplemented with 1,000 milligrams (mg) of calcium per day did have less bone loss than women who did not take a calcium supplement.[18] Supplementation may also be more beneficial for slowing bone loss when combined with an exercise program.[19]

In general, the most common advisable forms of calcium for supplementation are calcium carbonate, calcium phosphate, calcium gluconate, and calcium citrate. Previously it was accepted that calcium supplements required an acidic environment in order to dissolve and be absorbed by the body. However, recent research shows that the absorption of calcium has little to do with acidity or even solubility of the calcium source. As people age they generally absorb calcium less efficiently, but this probably is not due to decreased gastric acid production. Calcium carbonate was particularly singled out as requiring an acidic environment for absorption, but it is now known that even people with no stomach acid production have normal absorption if the supplement is taken with meals.[20] Calcium phosphate is found in dairy products and some supplements. Calcium gluconate is absorbed by most people. However, it has less calcium per weight than some of the other calcium supplements. Calcium citrate has been touted because it requires less of an acidic environment for dissolution, but as noted above, this is probably irrelevant to absorption.

Bonemeal and dolomite as nutritional supplements should be avoided. *Dairy Council Digest* has noted that those supplements may have other toxic ingredients such as lead and toxic metals.

Many people also use antacids as a calcium supplement. But some of the products contain aluminum, which can leach the calcium out of the bones, causing it to be excreted.

Food Sources of Calcium

Sources include dairy products, soybean products, green leafy vegetables, canned salmon with the bones, mackerel, sardines, and raisins.

Recommendations

The RDA for calcium is 800 mg for women 25 and over; the RDA for both pregnant and lactating women is 1,000 mg. Worldwide the recommended range varies from 400 to 1,000 mg per day. When calcium supplements are used, taking calcium carbonate at mealtimes is advisable for optimal absorption.[21]

Woman's Guide Suggestion

Under the age of 40, supplement with 1,000 to 1,500 mg of calcium daily; over that age, supplement with 1,500 to 2,000 mg daily. Women on estrogen replacement therapy/hormone replacement therapy (ERT/HRT) supplement with 1,200 to 1,500 mg daily.

Antagonists

Low levels of estrogen (after menopause) increase calcium loss. Red meats, alcohol, and foods with oxalic acid (a poisonous organic acid) impair the absorption of calcium.

Sources of oxalic acid are beet greens, spinach, rhubarb, chard, and almonds. Anticoagulants, antiseizure medication, and extended use of cortisone put women at a higher risk of osteoporosis. Higher phosphorus intake, caffeine products, tobacco, diets extremely high in fiber and carbonated beverages, and inactivity may interfere with calcium absorption.

Toxicity

No adverse side effects have been reported with intakes of calcium as high as 2,500 mg per day. One exception is an increase in the incidence of urinary stones in males.[22]

Warning

If you have kidney stones, kidney disease, or heart disease, check with your doctor before supplementing with calcium. Calcium reduces the amount of iron absorption.[23]

11

CHROMIUM

PRIMARY FUNCTIONS

Regulation of glucose metabolism
Synthesis of fatty acids and cholesterol
Protein transport
Lowers LDL and raises HDL blood levels
May protect against coronary artery disease

The mineral chromium has been shown to be helpful in regulation of glucose metabolism, and deficiency results in insulin resistance.[1] Individuals with some types of hypoglycemia (low blood sugar) have shown improvement in laboratory indices as well as in subjective symptoms, especially chilliness, after chromium supplementation.[2] It is thought that these represent cases of chromium deficiency. Supplementation will generally not correct glucose metabolism diseases such as diabetes. Trivalent chromium can lower the blood levels of ***low-density lipoproteins*** (LDL, "bad cholesterol") because high levels are associated with increased risk of heart disease and raise the ***high-density lipoproteins*** (HDL, "good cholesterol").[3] Low levels of chromium have also been associated with higher risk of coronary heart disease.[4] Some suspicions have been raised recently that the association between alcohol consumption and reduced rates of heart disease may actually be due to the chromium content of yeast-fermented alcoholic beverages, not the alcohol content.

Chromium concentrations in body tissues decrease with age, and the parallel with age-related glucose intolerance may not be coincidental. Presently no accurate technique is readily available to determine chromium status in an individual; therefore, it is difficult to determine the necessary chromium requirement. Total body stores do not correlate with serum (blood) or urine levels, and hair analysis is an unreliable indicator of chromium status in a given individual. Presently chromium deficiencies are best diagnosed in hindsight; that is, if a patient improves with supplementation, a retroactive diagnosis of chromium deficiency is made.

Chromium is a mineral found in the soil, and chromium-poor soil results in chromium-deficient foods. Processing foods and milling grains result in decreased amounts of chromium in the diet. Chromium losses are also exacerbated by strenuous exercise, pregnancy, infection, and stress.[5]

Food Sources of Chromium

Brewer's yeast is very high in chromium. However, care must be taken to be sure that the supplement is authentic brewer's yeast, as other sources (baker's yeast, etc.) do not contain significant amounts of chromium.[6] Other foods with chromium are wheat germ, whole grains, brown rice, beans, cheese, beer, and meat.

Recommendations

The RDA places a safe and adequate intake of chromium at 50 to 200 micrograms (mcg). Recently chromium picolinate has been highly touted as a supplement, but some authorities doubt that it is superior to the less expensive chromium chloride or brewer's yeast.

Woman's Guide Suggestion

Under the age of 40, supplement with 80 mcg daily; with 100 mcg daily after age 40.

Antagonists

The processing of grains removes most of the chromium. Teflon-coated utensils and cookware other than stainless steel may reduce the amount of chromium in food.

Toxicity

The toxic levels of chromium are unknown except in mining and industrial settings. Industrial toxicity is caused by a different class of chromium compounds than are found in food or used for supplementation.

12 COPPER

PRIMARY FUNCTIONS

Keeps blood vessels elastic
Needed for formation of elastin and collagen
Functions as an iron oxidizer
Essential for proper functioning of vitamin C

Copper is an important iron oxidizer, preventing free-radical formation (see Chapter 2). This helps prevent fats from becoming rancid or oxidizing,[1] which may be significant; it has been suggested that high iron blood levels may increase the risk of heart disease. (See Chapter 15.)

Elevated levels of copper have been discovered in patients with many different forms of cancer, including cancer of the female reproductive organs, bladder, large bowel, and stomach.[2]

Other researchers suspect that an increased risk of specific cancers may be associated with high copper and low zinc levels. In one study of 73 women hospitalized for suspected gynecological tumors, a correlation was found between the copper/zinc serum levels and tumor malignancies. The serum copper/zinc ratio was significantly higher in the malignant tumors than in the 48 benign growths. It was suggested that the copper/zinc ratio may be a marker for malignant tumors.[3] (See Chapter 22.)

The amount of copper we ingest in our daily diets is dependent on the amount of copper in the soil where the foods were grown and the animals were grazed. The copper is absorbed by plants, ingested by animals, and ultimately consumed by people.

Food Sources of Copper

Sources include kidneys, shellfish, legumes, liver, nuts, bran, soybeans, and wheat germ.

Antagonists

Ascorbic acid inhibits copper absorption.[4] Copper works in conjunction with both zinc and vitamin C; high levels of either zinc or vitamin C will lower copper levels. Intravenous feeding commonly causes copper deficiencies.

Recommendations

The RDA subcommittee has stated that a safe, adequate intake of copper is between 1.5 and 3 milligrams (mg) per day.[5]

Woman's Guide Suggestion

Supplement with 2 mg of copper daily.

Toxicity

Copper toxicity is rare in the United States. Most U.S. diets usually do not contain more than 5 mg per day, with an occasional high of 10 mg per day.

Warning

People with Wilson's disease (a disorder of copper metabolism) should not take copper supplements without consulting a physician.

13

FLUORIDE

PRIMARY FUNCTIONS

Increases bone density
Prevents osteoporosis-related fractures
Prevents dental decay

A fluoride is any binary compound of fluorine with another element. Although minute traces are found in all tissues, fluoride is found mostly in the bones and teeth, and it helps in their formation and strengthening. Fluoride is frequently added to public water supplies or applied directly to teeth to prevent dental decay. It also reduces the acid levels in saliva, which lowers the risk of tooth decay.

Since the 1960s numerous studies have supported the position that fluoride supplementation increases bone density and decreases the rate of fracture in osteoporotic bone disease. Some researchers analyzed populations living in areas with water supplies having high or low fluoride concentrations. Others dealt with daily supplementation with oral sodium fluoride. Lower rates of vertebral and hip fractures were seen in populations with higher fluoride levels.[1] Because of this evidence, sodium fluoride has become one of the commonly used treatments for osteoporosis.

However, a study done at Mayo Clinic and Henry Ford Hospital found that sodium fluoride increases bone density but does not decrease the rate of bone fracture. It has been known for years that high levels of fluoride cause a dense but brittle bone condition called *fluorosis*. However, there are criticisms of the study based on methodology, specifically the high dosage of fluoride administered and the particular form of calcium supplement used. Calcium carbonate was used as the calcium supplement, even though it is one of the more poorly absorbed calcium sources. The study is very controversial among researchers, but it does raise the question of whether bone density is a true risk indicator of osteoporosis.[2]

Food Sources of Fluoride

Fluoride is found in tea, drinking water, and fish eaten with their bones.

Recommendations

The estimated safe and adequate intake is 1.5 to 4.0 milligrams (mg) per day. The Food and Nutrition Board recommends that fluoride be added to the water supply if the levels are less than .7 mg per liter.

Woman's Guide Suggestion

There is enough fluoride in foods and the water supply that supplementation is not necessary.

Antagonists

Aluminum cooking vessels can reduce fluoride availability.

Toxicity

Twenty to 80 mg per day of fluoride can cause toxicity. Two to 8 mg per liter of fluoride in drinking water can cause mottling (spotting) of children's teeth. Toxic problems can sometimes occur in adults at 50 mg per day for several months. This is a dosage commonly used to treat osteoporosis, so a watchful eye for side effects is warranted.[3]

Warning

In children, tooth mottling often unexpectedly occurs due to the combined intakes of fluoride from a fluoridated water supply, a fluoride supplement from the child's pediatrician, and the large amounts ingested by swallowing lots of tasty fluoride toothpaste.

14

IODINE

PRIMARY FUNCTIONS

Metabolism of fats
Necessary for proper thyroid function
May reduce fibrocystic breast conditions

Iodine is turned into iodide in the body and has a significant role in the functioning of the thyroid gland. Iodine helps regulate metabolism, energy levels, and the burning of fat.

Researchers in Canada and the United States have used different dosages and regimens of iodine to treat fibrocystic breast disease. They have found that all of their patients were cyst free and 70 percent were pain free after four months of treatment; 95 percent of the women found relief of pain within a year. Long-standing fibrosis can take up to three years to eliminate.[1] Upon completion of testing four different types of iodine treatments on many women with fibrocystic disease, researchers concluded that molecular iodine (I_2) was the most beneficial.[2]

Food Sources of Iodine

Iodine is found in saltwater fish, kelp, garlic, sea salt, iodized table salt, mushrooms, soybeans, and summer squash.

Recommendations

The recommended daily allowance (RDA) for females ages 11 and up is 150 micrograms (mcg). The RDA for pregnant women is 175 mcg; for lactating women it is 200 mcg.

Woman's Guide Suggestion

Supplement with 150 mcg of iodine daily.

Antagonists

Brussels sprouts, cabbage, pears, spinach, and turnips may inhibit iodine absorption if eaten in large quantities.

Toxicity

In Japan, goiters (enlarged thyroid glands) have been induced by the consumption of large quantities of seaweed, which can contain 4.5 mg of iodine per gram dry weight. However, 1 to 2 mg of iodine per day have not resulted in any adverse physiological problems in healthy adults.[3]

15
IRON

PRIMARY FUNCTIONS

Production of hemoglobin and myoglobin
(hemoglobin's twin in muscle tissue)

Iron is a very controversial mineral. On one hand, it has been reported that up to 20 million Americans suffer from anemia,[1] much of it the result of iron deficiency. On the other hand, there is now a great concern that high levels of iron may be partly responsible for heart and liver disease. Iron is stored in the body by specialized proteins called *ferritin* and used as it is needed. As the level of stored iron increases, so does extra, free-floating iron. When the free iron comes in contact with oxygen, it accelerates chemical reactions in the body, causing oxidation damage to cell walls.[2]

Iron requirements are higher for women who are menstruating, pregnant, or lactating and lower for women postmenopausally. Menstruating women have iron stores of about 200–300 milligrams (mg). After menopause the iron stores (as well as the risk of heart disease) increase to approximately 800 mg—similar to that of men. R. B. Lauffer, researcher and author of *Iron Balance*, suggests that it would be best to keep the iron stores between 100 and 400 mg.[3] Iron stores can be reduced by regularly giving blood. Depending on your age, beware; food in the United States contains a great deal of iron fortification, and most multiple vitamins include iron.

Researchers have attempted to tie both high and low levels of iron to increased rates of infection, but the studies are controversial, and laboratory abnormalities appear to be more impressive than clinical evidence in humans. An exception should probably be made for iron supplementation in areas where malaria is a constant problem, where supplementation is followed by an increase in acute disease.[4]

Food Sources of Iron

Sources include red meats, fortified cereals and breads, fish, green leafy vegetables, poultry, and beans. Alcohol and vitamin C enhance iron absorption.

Recommendations

The recommended daily allowances (RDA) for women between the ages of 25 and 50 is 15 mg, and for women 50 and above the RDA is 10 mg. The RDA for pregnant women is 30 mg and for lactating women 15 mg.

Woman's Guide Suggestion

Under age 40, supplement with 15 mg of iron daily; at age 40 and older, supplement with 9 mg daily.

Antagonists

Phytates, complex organic phosphate salts found in unprocessed grains and some greens, prevent absorption of iron.

Toxicity

Iron intake between 25 and 75 mg per day has not caused problems in healthy adults. Taking 200 to 250 mg per kilogram (kg) of body weight in one dose can be lethal. Approximately 2,000 cases of iron poisoning occur yearly in the United States. These reported cases are mostly in children who take their parents' adult iron supplements.

Warning

High levels of iron postmenopausally have been suggested to increase the risk of heart disease. Inorganic iron can inhibit vitamin E absorption. A small population of people with *idiopathic hemochromatosis* is genetically at risk for iron overload. They absorb iron too efficiently from the intestines and can suffer from chronic iron toxicity, leading to heart and liver damage.

16

MAGNESIUM

PRIMARY FUNCTIONS

Involved in over 330 enzymatic reactions[1]
Bone formation and growth
Prevention of bone loss
Coronary artery relaxant
May prevent heart disease
Managing *preeclampsia* (a hypertensive disorder of pregnancy sometimes leading to convulsions), treating cardiac *arrythmias* (irregular heart beats),[2] and managing diabetes[3]

Magnesium plays a significant role in the formation and structure of bones. The body contains about 25 grams of magnesium, and 50–60 percent of that is in the bones.[4] People in the United States had a higher magnesium intake in their diets at the beginning of the century than they do presently. Today the U.S. diet contains less grain than it did in the past, and milling has removed most of the magnesium in the grain we do eat.[5]

Magnesium metabolism appears to change postmenopausally and after an ovariectomy (surgical removal of an ovary or ovaries). When the estrogen levels drop, an increased excretion of magnesium occurs. Estrogen restores the magnesium levels by increasing intestinal absorption. In a study based on the NHANES I, investigators looked at the serum magnesium levels of 224 pregnant women, 1,559 nonpregnant women taking birth control pills, 2,884 postmenopausal women between the ages of 50 and 74, and 4,145 nonpregnant women in a control group between the ages of 15 and 49. They found that pregnant women and women on the pill had reduced serum magnesium levels when compared to the control group. Postmenopausal women had the highest serum magnesium levels.[6]

Other researchers, examining the role of magnesium and bone loss, compared different estrogen and hormone replacement therapies used by postmenopausal women and compared those results to a control group. The data indicated that the women who took estrogen with a *progestogen* (a substance that acts like *progesterone*, a female hormone secreted by the ovary before ovulation) decreased their urinary excretion of magnesium.[7] Although the exact role of magnesium in bone loss is not clear, the researchers indicated that low levels of magnesium may be one of the factors that contribute to osteoporosis. They also suggested that the present recommended magnesium intake may be too low.

An interesting study that looked specifically at the relationship between magnesium and calcium followed postmenopausal women who were taking varied and different types of replacement therapies. Those who took 500 milligrams (mg) of calcium and 1,000 mg of magnesium reversed their bone loss. They showed a significant increase in bone mineral density within a year. Because the bulk of the research does not support calcium megadosing in the postmenopausal years, researchers suggested a change in the recommended daily allowance (RDA) levels of both calcium and magnesium. The authors proposed raising the magnesium levels to 1,000 mg per day and lowering the calcium levels to 500 mg per day.[8] Further research is being conducted with women not taking replacement therapies to see if they also have reduced bone loss with higher magnesium intakes.

Magnesium, vitamin D, phosphorus, sodium, potassium, manganese, and calcium all interact. The optimal ratios among these agents are not known, but a balance is assumed to be critical for bone formation and health. It is generally accepted that about a 1 to 3 ratio of magnesium to calcium be maintained. However, as pointed out above, some researchers are advocating the reverse of this ratio.

Interest also exists in magnesium's role in ischemic (coronary) heart disease, where blood flow to the heart muscle is reduced, usually because of a narrowing of the coronary arteries. Magnesium is important as a coronary artery relaxant, and it is necessary for normal cardiac electrical function. Many different heart problems have been attributed to magnesium deficiencies. Low levels of magnesium are associated with abnormal heart rhythms and sudden-death ischemic heart disease, and intravenous magnesium given to acute heart attack patients has shown reductions in death, arrhythmias, and heart failure. Reviews of epidemiological and geographical studies show that areas with low magnesium levels in the water and the soil have higher death rates from ischemic heart disease.[9]

Studies have been done on the prevalence of heart disease in geographic areas having hard or soft water supplies. Hard water has more calcium and magnesium than does soft water. Water softeners replace the calcium and magnesium with sodium. (High sodium levels may be a problem for some people.) Individuals who drink soft water were found to have lower levels of magnesium in their cardiac muscle. They also have a higher incidence of sudden-death ischemic heart disease.[10]

Food Sources of Magnesium

Sources include green vegetables, seafood, legumes, nuts, meats, and many dairy products. Most of the magnesium has been removed from processed grains.

Recommendations

The RDA for women over 25 is 280 mg. The RDA for pregnant women is 300 mg. The RDA for lactating women is 355 mg in the first six months and 340 mg from six months on. Magnesium gluconate is commonly used as a supplement.

Woman's Guide Suggestion

Under the age of 40, supplement with 400 to 600 mg of magnesium daily; at age 40 and after, supplement with 500 to 700 mg daily.

Antagonists

High levels of calcium can interfere with magnesium absorption. Diabetes, heart problems, alcoholism, cirrhosis, any trauma to the body, and any malabsorption problems can interfere with magnesium absorption.[11] Diuretics can inhibit magnesium absorption.

Toxicity

Presently there is no evidence that high levels of magnesium cause any serious problems, except as noted below in cases of heart or kidney disease.

Warning

Large doses of magnesium will work as a laxative. People with kidney problems or cardiac patients who have heart block should talk with their physicians before using a magnesium supplement.

17

MANGANESE

PRIMARY FUNCTIONS

Bone growth
Possible prevention of osteoporosis
Regulates production and release of insulin
Metabolizes fats and proteins
Nerve transmission
Production of mother's milk
Production of thyroxine (thyroid gland hormone)

Manganese is necessary for bone growth and may play a part in preventing osteoporosis. Recent studies on osteoporosis showed that women with the disease had manganese levels from 29 percent to 75 percent below that of controls.[1] Manganese absorption is a problem in that many high-manganese foods also contain agents that inhibit manganese absorption. Calcium supplementation (as for osteoporosis prevention) can also decrease manganese absorption from the diet.

Food Sources of Manganese

Manganese occurs in whole grains, nuts, vegetables, fruits, milk, meats, and eggs.

Recommendations

The recommended daily allowance (RDA) has a provisional level set between 2 and 5 milligrams (mg) per day.

Woman's Guide Suggestion

Supplement with 5 mg of manganese daily.

Antagonists

Large amounts of calcium, phosphorus, magnesium, and phytates (found in whole grains), tannins, and oxalic acids will inhibit absorption.

Toxicity

The only toxicity reported has been from environmental exposure rather than dietary.

Warning

Women with low manganese levels may be at risk for increased iron loss due to menstrual bleeding.[2]

18

Molybdenum

PRIMARY FUNCTIONS

Metabolizes fats
Has biochemical role in functioning of enzymes
Plays a role in iron utilization

Many researchers state that molybdenum supplementation is unnecessary unless food comes from soil deficient in the mineral. Individuals who have a deficiency in molybdenum may have an increased incidence of esophageal cancer.[1]

Food Sources of Molybdenum

Sources include milk, beans, breads, whole grains, legumes, and organ meats.

Recommendations

The recommended daily allowance (RDA) for a safe and adequate intake of molybdenum is 75 to 250 micrograms (mcg). The daily requirements of this element can be met in the daily diet. The public water supply usually provides 2 to 8 mcg daily.

Woman's Guide Suggestion

Supplement with 15 mcg of molybdenum daily.

Antagonists

Sulfate may inhibit the absorption of molybdenum. Molybdenum and copper in the intestinal tract form a compound that inhibits the absorption of both elements. This is modified by dietary sulfur.

Toxicity

Ten milligrams (mg) per day of molybdenum has produced toxic reactions. Copper loss in the urine has resulted from 0.54 mg per day.

19

PHOSPHORUS

PRIMARY FUNCTIONS

Formation of bones and teeth
Muscle contraction
Kidney functions
Nervous system transmission

Phosphorus is a part of every cell in the body but is especially necessary for the formation of bones and teeth. Approximately 85 percent of phosphorus is found in the bones. A balance between phosphorus and calcium intakes is very important. A less than 1 to 2 ratio of dietary calcium to phosphorus may cause a lowered calcium blood level. In some animal studies, a low calcium-to-phosphorus ratio leads to bone resorption.[1] People who consume little in the way of dairy products and green vegetables can have a calcium-to-phosphorus ratio as low as 1 to 4.

Foods Rich in Phosphorus

Phosphorus is contained in almost all foods but is very high in both sodas and red meats. Most "junk foods" are very high in phosphorus and should be avoided.

Recommendations

The recommended daily allowance (RDA) for women age 25 and above is 800 milligrams (mg). The RDA for pregnant and lactating women is 1,200 mg.

Woman's Guide Suggestion

Supplementation of phosphorus is not necessary, as adequate amounts of phosphorus are consumed in the diet.

Antagonists

Aluminum hydroxide, found in some antacids, inhibits absorption of phosphorus.

Toxicity

Phosphorus has no known toxic level. However, high levels causing calcium-to-phosphorus ratios less than 1 to 2 have resulted in bone resorption in animals.

Warning

Phosphorus levels in normal diets in the United States are not thought to be dangerous to humans, especially with adequate intake of calcium and vitamin D.[2]

20
POTASSIUM

PRIMARY FUNCTIONS

May reduce risk of strokes
Maintains good blood pressure
Needed for transmission of nerve impulses
Needed for proper muscle contraction

A ubiquitous element in virtually all living cells, potassium is a key constituent of the "internal ocean" of salts in which our tissues live. It is necessary in one way or another for almost any function of any tissue, but especially for nerve transmission and muscle contraction.

A 1987 study, done over a 12-year period, found that men and women who consumed a high potassium diet suffered fewer strokes. One extra serving of a fresh vegetable or fruit per day was associated with a 40 percent reduced risk of stroke-associated mortality.[1]

Recommendations

The National Research Council states that the minimum potassium requirement is between 1,600 milligrams (mg) and 2,000 mg per day. However, ingesting 3,500 mg per day may have a beneficial effect on hypertension (high blood pressure). The council recommends an additional intake of fruits and vegetables. No recommendation is given for increased levels for pregnant or lactating women.[2]

Woman's Guide Suggestion

Supplementation of potassium is not necessary, since adequate amounts are consumed in the diet.

Food Sources of Potassium

Potassium is found in fruits, vegetables, fresh meats, legumes, fish, and whole grains.

Antagonists

Processed foods often have decreased potassium and increased sodium. Alcohol and coffee cause potassium loss.

Toxicity

Eighteen grams a day can cause acute intoxication and death by *cardiac arrest* (the heart stops pumping blood). Lesser amounts usually harmless to someone with normal kidneys may result quickly in fatal *hyperkalemia* (high potassium blood levels) in persons with chronic kidney failure.

Warning

Some diuretics and extended periods of vomiting or diarrhea will deplete potassium. As noted above, increased intake of potassium is dangerous to persons with renal (kidney) failure.

21
SELENIUM

PRIMARY FUNCTIONS

Acts as antioxidant
May reduce risk of heart attack and heart disease
May reduce risk of cancers
Protects against metal poisoning
Synergistic with vitamin E

Selenium is a trace mineral in the soil. The selenium content of fruits, vegetables, and grains varies depending on the selenium levels of the soil in which they grew. Reportedly the most selenium-poor soil in the United States is around the Great Lakes, in most of the east coast, and in the west coast. These areas are also reported to have the highest incidence of breast cancer.[1]

Research studies have shown a relationship between low selenium levels and an increased risk of myocardial infarction. One study, which examined 84 patients with heart problems and 84 without, found significantly lower serum selenium levels in patients with myocardial infarction. The patients had low levels of selenium in their toenails, which indicated that the low selenium levels preceded the heart attacks.[2]

A comparison of people with high and low selenium blood levels in China encountered many fewer cases of esophageal, stomach, and liver cancer among subjects with higher levels of selenium.[3]

A Finnish four-year prospective study ending in 1980 determined that low selenium and low vitamin E levels were significantly associated with increased cancer death rates in men.[4]

Another study compared two groups of 30 healthy post-menopausal women from both Finland and Japan. Compared to Japan, Finland has a high incidence of coronary heart disease, breast cancer, and endometrial (uterine lining) cancer. Finland is also a selenium-poor country in comparison to Japan. The researchers compared selenium, vitamin A, vitamin E, and cholesterol levels. The findings showed no differences in serum vitamin A levels, but the Finns had higher vitamin E and cholesterol and lower serum selenium levels than did the Japanese.[5] It was suggested that these vitamin and selenium variations could account for the differences in risk of heart disease and cancer for these two countries.

The exact relationship between selenium and vitamin E is unknown, but the two are interdependent. One of the above studies found a synergistic relationship between low selenium and vitamin E levels as a predictive marker for cancer death.[6] In addition, a few deficiency diseases can be reversed by therapy with either selenium or vitamin E.[7]

Selenium has also been shown to protect the body against silver, mercury, and cadmium toxicity.[8]

Food Sources of Selenium

Selenium occurs in seafood, liver, kidneys, grains, chicken, egg yolk, mushrooms, and garlic.

Recommendations

The recommended daily allowance (RDA) for women over 25 is 55 micrograms (mcg). The RDA is 65 mcg for pregnant women and 75 mcg for lactating women.

Woman's Guide Suggestion

Supplement with 50 mcg of selenium daily.

Toxicity

Chronic intake of 5 milligrams per day has caused hair loss and fingernail changes.[9]

22
ZINC

PRIMARY FUNCTIONS

Required trace element of DNA and RNA
Needed for growth and sexual development
Required for proper alcohol metabolism

Zinc is needed by virtually all plants and animals. It is a critical component for the growth of children and for their sexual development. Zinc is important during pregnancy and lactation and is a necessary nutrient for fetal development. Zinc deficiency has been associated with abnormalities in taste, poor wound healing, skin lesions, and immune dysfunction.[1]

Assessing zinc status in people is difficult. Zinc deficiency is often covert until it results in an obvious problem. Researchers have shown that postmenopausal women showed no significant change in serum zinc levels even after four months of relative zinc deprivation. This is despite the fact that more-sophisticated assays of zinc-dependent function indicated a decrease in activity that was corrected by zinc supplementation. The conclusion was that zinc levels in the blood may not be a reliable indicator of deficiency states. An overt problem due to zinc deficiency may appear before detection is possible, especially in the elderly, who are more prone to zinc deficiencies than younger people.[2]

Alcoholics generally have low levels of zinc, which may be due to an inadequate diet or to alcohol inhibiting zinc absorption. This may be a compounded problem since low zinc levels decrease the body's ability to metabolize alcohol, resulting in prolonged exposure to high alcohol levels and increased tissue damage.[3]

Estrogen in pre- and postmenopausal women lowers zinc levels in the blood. It also raises the copper to levels similar to those seen in pregnant women. Some researchers have concluded that a progestogen should be added to postmenopausal hormone treatments to balance the copper-to-zinc ratios.[4]

Food Sources of Zinc

Sources include oysters, meats, poultry, and some vegetables. Breast milk and zinfandel wine enhance the bioavailability of zinc.

Recommendations

The recommended daily allowance (RDA) for women 25 and older is 12 milligrams (mg). The RDA for pregnant women is 15 mg. The RDA for lactating women is 19 mg the first six months and then drops to 16 mg.

Woman's Guide Suggestion

Under the age of 40, supplement with 20 mg of zinc daily. After age 40, supplement with 30 mg daily.

Antagonists

Phytates, high-fiber diets, tin, oxalate, copper, and possibly high phosphorus intake inhibit zinc absorption. Vegetarians, athletes, and dieters tend to have lower levels of zinc. It appears that the bioavailability of zinc is very dependent on the total diet, and all of its antagonists are not clearly understood.

Toxicity

Zinc in the amount of 18.5 mg per day has been shown to create an impairment of copper metabolism. Large doses of 2 grams or more can acutely cause nausea and vomiting. Chronically taking more than 10 times the RDA can result in many problems.[5]

III
Topics of Prime Concern to Women

23
Bones

Bones have 70 percent mineral and 30 percent organic components. The organic matter is mostly collagen, and the minerals are largely calcium and phosphorus salts. There are two types of bone tissue: cortical and trabecular. *Cortical bone tissue* forms the outer shell of the bone and is mostly found in the shafts of long bones such as the humerus (arm) and femur (thigh). *Trabecular bone* is the porous bone tissue mostly found in the vertebrae (backbone), the flat bones (face, pelvis, skull), and the distal (far) ends of the long bones. However, in many locations throughout the body, bones contain both cortical and trabecular bone in varying proportion.

Bones go through a very regular growth pattern consisting of stages of bone resorption and bone remodeling. This resorption and rebuilding is called bone "turnover." The first stage of resorption begins with *osteoclasts* (specialized bone demolition cells) dissolving some of the bone tissue and leaving an excavated or dug-out area in the bone. In the next stage, the *osteoblasts* (bone construction cells) begin rebuilding a collagen framework for new bone in the excavated areas. The osteoblasts continue rebuilding until mineralization of the bone takes place; then they go into a resting stage. Up to 10 percent of the bone throughout the body is actively involved in these different stages at the same time. The entire resorption-remodeling process takes about 100 days to complete. Under the best of conditions in adulthood the bone remodeling and bone resorption are equal to one another, and no net bone loss occurs until menopause.

In a normal, healthy person, until the approximate age of 35–40 the cortical bones keep developing to reach peak mass. The trabecular bones reach their peak mass at about the age of 25–30 years.[1] In early adulthood the bones stop building and may begin to decline. Generally, a woman does not have any significant bone loss until menopause unless she has specific health problems, develops *amenorrhea* (stops menstruating) due to excessive exercise, has anorexia nervosa, or does not eat properly. Any of these conditions can lead to an increased risk of osteoporosis.

Bone loss becomes problematic at menopause. Hormonal changes accelerate bone loss for approximately one decade. At that point the bone loss returns to a slower, age-related loss rate similar to that of men. At about the age of 40 a woman will lose approximately 0.3 percent to 0.4 percent of her total bone mass each year. After menopause the bone loss may accelerate up to 2 percent to 3 percent each year.[2]

Osteoporosis is a disease characterized by a reduction of bone mass that leads to bone fracture(s). Both cortical and trabecular bones become weakened and are unable to withstand the stresses of normal daily life. Microscopically the bones take on the appearance of Swiss cheese. Some women develop a dowager's hump. The spinal vertebrae become so porous that their collapse creates the characteristic pronounced hump on the upper back.

Worldwide, osteoporosis is more of a problem in urban, highly industrialized areas.[3] It is less prevalent in locations where the diets contain whole grains, fish, tofu, and seaweed. Except for the women who are on estrogen supplementation, all postmenopausal women experience higher rates of bone loss than other healthy people; it is not known why some women develop actual osteoporosis and some do not. Hormone supplementation reduces the amount of calcium lost and delays the menopausal bone loss.[4] But replacement therapy is not without risk. (See Chapter 25.)

Osteoporosis affects approximately 20 million people, mostly women, in the United States each year. The disease results in approximately 1.2 million fractures yearly. One-third of all women will have fractures by age 65, and one-third of women will have a fractured hip by extreme old age.[5] Although fewer than 2 percent of women over age 65 will die from osteoporosis-related hip fractures,[6] the sickness, pain, and related expense of fractures are staggering. The mortality rate for people in the first year after a hip fracture is 12 percent to 20 percent higher than for people without fractures;[7] the estimated total annual cost for caring for people with osteoporosis, both directly and indirectly, is between $7 billion and $12 billion.[8]

Osteoporosis has been categorized as either primary (type I) or secondary (type II). *Type I osteoporosis* affects women after menopause. It mainly affects trabecular bone, which leads to many spinal fractures. An estimated 5 percent to 10 percent of women get osteoporosis marked by a spinal fracture within the first 15 to 20 years after menopause.[9] *Type II osteoporosis* generally affects women over 70 years old. It is an age-related bone loss and affects both cortical and trabecular bones.[10]

Postmenopausal women are also at the highest risk for requiring major dental work. Osteoporosis plays a large role in deterioration of the teeth and jaw bone structure, which makes dental work very difficult.[11] One source stated that approximately 40 percent of women will have lost their teeth by age 60. The author did not resolve the question of whether the loss of teeth was due to poor dental care, osteoporosis, or a combination of the two.[12]

Exercise has been shown to play a large role both in bone growth and in retarding bone loss. Weight-bearing exercise, weight lifting, aerobic dance, walking, and exercise that involves full-range motions have been shown to be the most beneficial.[13] It appears that 20 to 45 minutes of moderate exercise such as dancing, aerobics, and jogging is effective in helping to maintain bone density.[14] A new study of over 200 women indicates that walking over a mile daily as regular exercise is associated with a greater overall bone density. However, although walking appeared to reduce the rate of bone loss from the legs, it had no effect on bone loss from other areas of the skeleton.[15] A different group concluded, after a two-year follow-up of 65 postmenopausal women not on estrogen or hormone replacement therapy, that non-weight-bearing exercises were ineffective in reducing vertebral bone loss.[16] However, falls and the fractures they cause are major causes of death in elderly women in the United States. Any exercise that increases muscle tone, balance, and agility will also help to reduce the risk in falling.[17]

Exercise also is known to help cardiovascular health, gastrointestinal health, and psychological health. Yet the benefits gained from exercise are short lived and reversible;[18] when physical activity and stress on bone and muscles are eliminated, the bone mineral density decreases.[19] People who are immobile or bedridden for prolonged periods have a large loss of bone.[20] Exercise needs to be a part of a lifelong routine.

Studies on the value of calcium supplementation after menopause are conflicting.[21] However, in general, the majority of researchers recommend that young women consume a diet high in calcium, that premenopausal women supplement their diets with 1,000 milligrams (mg) of calcium per day, that postmenopausal women not on estrogen or hormone replacement therapy supplement their diets with 1,500 mg of calcium per day, and that postmenopausal women on estrogen or hormone replacement therapy supplement their diets with 1,000 mg of calcium per day. Other experts on calcium metabolism, pointing to the low risks of calcium supplementation, the devastating effects of osteoporosis, and the high intake of calcium in the diets of aboriginal men and primates, advocate considerably larger amounts. (See Chapter 10.)

The major factors in maintaining bone health in premenopausal women are listed here in order of decreasing importance: active ovarian function, physical activity, calcium intake, body size, low alcohol consumption, and a lack of cigarette smoking. In postmenopausal women, the factors that proved most important are calcium intake and physical activity.[22]

Many factors put a woman at higher risk of osteoporosis:

Fair complexion
Old age
Early or surgical menopause (reduction of estrogen)
Amenorrhea (reduction of estrogen)
A thin body build (below 15 percent body fat is high risk)
Caucasian or Asian race
Family history
Drugs (corticosteroids, thyroxine, etc.)
Low-calcium diet
Smoking cigarettes
High alcohol consumption
Physical inactivity
Specific health problems
Low nutrient absorption in postmenopausal women[23]

In summary, for good bone health, women should:

- Achieve as much bone mass as possible before age 35
- Eat a well-balanced diet high in calcium
- Supplement with calcium, vitamin D, magnesium, boron, manganese, and phosphorus
- Take regular exercise, both aerobic and weight-bearing
- Possibly take an estrogen supplement
- Be aware of medications that reduce bone density, such as steroids, anticoagulants, and anticonvulsants
- Eat foods high in acids (citrus, tomatoes, cranberry juice, vinegars, etc.), which improve calcium absorption
- Avoid carbonated soda beverages, as these contain high levels of phosphate and interfere with calcium absorption

Bone mineral density can be measured by different methods. Four are commonly used: tomography, both single photon and dual-photon absorptiometry, and the newer technique of dual-energy x-ray absorptiometry. In general, the tests use a small amount of radiation exposure, less than 5 millirem per study, and are accurate to within 1 percent or 2 percent. The bone measurements can be used to establish a baseline, determine risk, prescribe treatment, and evaluate treatment effectiveness. The bone measurement test costs approximately $200.

After menopause, a bone density study should be done on women with a family history of osteoporosis or any history of disease or medication associated with rapid bone loss. The study should be repeated at three- to five-year intervals. Yearly bone density studies are recommended in patients being treated with calcitonin or biophosphonates for established osteoporosis (see below).

Osteoporosis therapy is evolving rapidly. A few years ago no treatment was available. Now, along with calcium supplementation, there are estrogen (the most commonly used agent), calcitonin, and the biophosphonates. Calcitonin, available in the United States in its injectable form, has represented a major advance in therapy. Currently the only FDA-approved treatment for osteoporosis, it will increase bone strength as well as diminish the pain of vertebral compression fractures. Another class of drugs, the biophosphonates, also shows great promise. One example of this class is Didronel®[24] (etidronate disodium), originally used to treat *hypercalcemia* (high calcium blood levels) associated with malignancies. It also increases bone density and thus is helpful with osteoporosis. Other biophosphonates are now under investigation as well. In addition to these, insulin-like growth factors and slow-release fluoride look like hopeful future therapies.

An effective osteoporosis treatment must increase bone density, decrease fracture rate, and improve quality of life. More agents fitting this description will be available in the next few decades. Already today osteoporosis is preventable and, even in severe cases, treatable.

24
CANCER

Cancer is a number of different diseases grouped together by their characteristic behavior: abnormal cells grow in an uncontrolled manner and spread. Cancer is caused by diverse influences, including internal and external factors. Many of these factors are unknown, but the known include various chemicals, radiation, viruses, hormones, immune dysfunctions, and individual genetic predispositions.

Cancers from six sites represent the majority of cancer cases and cause half the deaths due to cancer. These sites are the colon and rectum, lung, breast, uterus, oral cavity, and skin. Many cancers can be prevented by avoiding tobacco, sun exposure, excess dietary fat, and other environmental factors known to be carcinogenic. Approximately 30 percent of all deaths due to cancer are related to tobacco use; this number translates into one in six deaths in the United States each year. Diet is suspected to be responsible for 35 percent of deaths due to cancer,[1] and most skin cancers are caused by excessive sun exposure.

Many cancers can be cured if they are found and treated early. Regular cancer checkups, including a mammogram, Pap test, and rectal exam, are important.

Cancer Facts 1992[2]

• The estimated number of new cancers in all sites for women was 565,000. The estimated number of deaths for women from cancer in all sites was 245,000. Not included in the above total were an estimated 20,000 new carcinomas in situ (noninvasive) of the breast in women and 55,000 carcinomas in situ of the uterine cervix. Also, nonmelanoma skin cancers were not included in the estimations. More than 600,000 cases of nonmelanoma skin cancers in both men and women are reported each year, with the vast majority being curable. Basal and squamous cell skin cancers have the highest cure rates.

• The estimated number of new cases of breast cancer in women was 180,000. One in nine women will get breast cancer in her lifetime. There has been a 3 percent yearly increase in breast cancer since 1980.

• The estimated number of new cases of melanoma in women was 15,000. There has been a reported 4 percent increase yearly in melanomas since 1973. Melanomas can be deadly and must be treated in the early stages.

• The estimated number of new cancers of digestive organs in women was 113,900.

• The estimated number of new genital or reproductive organ cancers in women was 71,500.

• The estimated number of new cases of respiratory system cancers in women was 70,000, of which 66,000 were lung cancers. *Note:* Today more women die of lung cancer than of breast cancer.

Breast Cancer

Many breast cancers are caused by a specific gene, called BRCA1, on the long arm of chromosome 17. It can be inherited from either father or mother and causes a good portion of breast cancers arising before age 40. The one woman in 200 who carries this gene has an 80 percent to 90 percent chance of developing breast cancer, as well as an increased chance of ovarian cancer.[3] Genetic counseling and testing can identify these high-risk women; many may choose to have prophylactic mastectomies rather than to sit on a time bomb that has an 85 percent chance of going off.[4]

Dietary fat and the use of hormones have been examined to determine their roles in promoting cancer. The studies have proven to be very controversial (see Chapter 25). The methodology in the studies has been questioned. It is very difficult to control for the number of variables that exist and for individual differences. These factors make the determination of cause and effect extremely difficult.

It is interesting to compare various countries' lifestyles and their rates of cancer and mortality. The United States has one of the highest rates of breast cancer in the world. Japan has about one-fourth the U.S. rate of breast cancer and has the longest life expectancy in the world. The two countries have many dietary differences. The traditional Japanese consume about 11 percent of their calories as fat. They generally eat a low-meat, high-fiber, heavily fish-based diet.[5] People in the United States consume about 40 percent of their calories from fat and eat a high-meat, low-fiber diet. Research has shown that women whose diets are high in fiber and low in fat have lower estrogen levels than do women whose diets are low in fiber and high in fat. A study of postmenopausal women found that meat-eating women in Boston had a 300 percent higher serum level of natural estrogen than did Asian immigrants living in Hawaii. Estrogen levels were also found to be 30 percent to 75 percent higher in premenopausal meat-eating women than in the Asian immigrants.[6] When Japanese women adopt a western diet similar to that of the United States, their rate of breast cancer increases to that found in the United States.[7]

However, in 1976 a longitudinal study began called the Harvard Nurses Health Study. More than 120,000 women were monitored over a decade, using successive questionnaires covering multiple areas including estrogen use, smoking habits, eating habits, and overall health. The results indicated that the risk of breast cancer due to a diet with over 50 percent fat was no higher than that from a diet with as much as 29 percent fat.[8] Peter Greenwald, a cancer specialist at the National Institutes of Health, points out that the nurses study only looked at women whose fat intake was 27 percent to 50 percent of their total caloric intake. It may be necessary to reduce the amount of fat intake below 20 percent or 25 percent of total calories to see a reduction in the risk of breast cancer. The nurses study did not look at these lower fat intakes.[9] However, the Harvard School of Public Health, in a 1992 conference, reported an association between *trans*-fatty acid intake and breast cancer in a review of 85,000 nurses.[10] (See Chapter 28 for a discussion of *trans*-fatty acids.)

Recently attention has turned away from fats to another long-standing suspect: estrogen exposure. The length of time spent bathing the breast tissues in a cyclically fluctuating estrogen environment appears to affect the risk of breast cancer. Thus early ***menarche*** (first menstruation) and late menopause both have been associated with increased risk. This may be one of the reasons for the disparate rates of breast cancer in the United States and in countries such as China. Presently Chinese women begin to menstruate at the age of 17, just as North American women did 200 years ago. Today women in the United States begin to menstruate at a mean age of 12.8 years. The sustained high hormonal levels associated with pregnancy, however, appear to be protective against later breast cancer development—so much so that a woman who has her first child at age 20 has half the breast cancer risk of a woman who waits until 30.[11]

Estrogen replacement therapy and hormone replacement therapy cause concern and controversy over the extent of the increased risk of cancer. A Swedish study of 23,244 women found a link between estrogen therapy and breast cancer. It found that women doubled their risk of breast cancer after using estradiol for a nine-year period. Women who took estradiol with a progestin (progesterone-like agent) increased the risk of breast cancer fourfold.

This study has been criticized on several grounds. First, the estrogen used in the study was estradiol, a form of estrogen different from and more potent than that commonly used in the United States; the dosages of estrogen used are in question. Second, the progestins used in the study were also different forms and dosages from those used in the United States.[12] Critics thus maintain that the results of the Swedish study cannot be extrapolated to estrogen replacement therapy or hormone replacement therapy in the United States.

The researchers in the Harvard Nurses Health Study found a 35 percent to 36 percent increase in breast cancer in women who took estrogen, compared to those who did not.[13] Others have concluded that women who take estrogen replacement therapy have a 40 percent increased risk of breast cancer over women who have never used estrogen. Women on the birth control pill have a 50 percent increased risk of breast cancer while on the pill. The rates of cancer drop back to baseline once the estrogen is stopped. It is suspected that estrogen may *promote* the growth of existing tumors rather than initiate that growth.[14] In Japan the birth control pill is not available to women; it has not been approved as safe by Japan's equivalent of the U.S. Food and Drug Administration.

Still others found that, although women who used estrogen had an increased risk of breast cancer, the estrogen users who developed cancer had a 10 percent to 20 percent lower risk of cancer death than nonusers who developed breast cancer. These findings have been attributed to the fact that women using estrogen are screened more closely and the tumors are found earlier than in nonusers.[15]

The cancer risks of using hormone replacement therapy are unknown. One hypothesis is that the risk of breast cancer is increased by estrogen alone and is increased further when a progestogen is added. It is suggested that estrogen plus a progestogen increases stimulation of cell division more than just estrogen alone. This viewpoint, however, is disputed by some researchers. Breast cancer risk increases with age, late menopause, early menarche, and obesity after menopause and is decreased premenopausally with obesity.[16]

Prevention

See Chapter 28, "Food," for cancer prevention recommendations by the American Cancer Society, the American Institute of Cancer Research, and the U.S. Department of Health and Human Services. See individual chapters on the antioxidant nutrients for their associations with reduced cancer risks.

25

ESTROGEN AND HORMONE REPLACEMENT THERAPIES

In 1989 more than 3.5 million women were taking estrogens for menopausal problems.[1] Women taking *estrogen replacement therapy (ERT)* or *hormone replacement therapy (HRT)*, a combination of estrogen and a progestogen (a substance that mimics the effects of progesterone), need to know and understand the unresolved issues and concerns about these treatments. ERT and HRT are relatively new therapies, and the research studies are incomplete. Never before have such a large proportion of aging women taken drugs to prolong a hormonal state similar to that of younger women. This type of therapy offers both benefits and risks. Some of the consequences may be yet unknown.[2]

Listed below is a sampling of recommendations made by various physicians and researchers.

- Hormone therapy should be given to premenopausal women who have had a hysterectomy or who have or are at high risk for coronary heart disease.[3]
- Short-term therapy with a gradual withdrawal is bene-

ficial for menopausal problems. Long-term therapy or life-long therapy may be necessary for urogenital (vaginal and urinary tract) problems.[4] (See Chapter 31.)

- Hormone therapy should be recommended for women who have had a hysterectomy, have coronary heart disease, or are at risk for coronary heart disease. However, the benefits of HRT are not clearly understood, and the risk of increasing breast cancer is a concern. More research is needed.[5]
- Hormone therapy is clearly indicated for women who have lost their ovaries before the age of 40, have a strong history of osteoporosis, or have a history of long-term steroid use.[6]

Women have differing physical and emotional needs and risks. Each needs to be aware of the pros and cons of taking ERT or HRT and make a personal decision depending on her particular health needs. It is a difficult and confusing decision to make because of the lack of information about the long-term effects and because of the range of opinion concerning treatments. Various authorities have widely divergent opinions concerning the use of replacement therapies. The U.S. Food and Drug Administration (FDA) has approved Premarin estrogen therapy for hot flashes, atrophic vaginitis (thinning and drying changes in the vagina), osteoporosis, low estrogen states due to removal or failure of the ovaries, uterine bleeding due to hormonal imbalance, and palliation (alleviation of symptoms rather than cure) in cases of advanced breast cancer.[7] In 1990 the FDA's Fertility and Maternal Health Drugs Advisory Committee judged that replacement therapy with Premarin may have value in reducing women's risks of heart and blood vessel diseases. The FDA, however, has not yet made a determination on this recommendation.[8] Note that although there are several different estrogen preparations used in the United States, their effects are not identical and neither are their indicated uses.

ERT

Contraindications for ERT and HRT

1. Active cancer of the breast, uterus, or ovary or history of recent (less than five years) cancer of the breast, uterus, or ovary
2. Liver disease, including hepatitis
3. Undiagnosed vaginal bleeding
4. Pregnancy (to avoid possible birth defects)
5. Active deep-vein *thrombophlebitis* (inflammation of a vein with formation of a blood clot)
6. Uncontrolled high blood pressure
7. Diseases affected negatively by increased fluid retention

Advantages of ERT

1. Eliminates hot flashes and night sweats (profuse nocturnal sweating with a variety of causes, including hot flashes)
2. Reduces loss of calcium from the bones, lowering the risk of osteoporosis
3. Prevents drying and shrinking of vaginal and urinary tract tissues
4. Reduces heart disease by increasing the production of high-density lipoprotein (HDL), or good cholesterol, and decreasing the level of low-density lipoprotein (LDL), or bad cholesterol

Disadvantages of ERT

1. When unopposed by progesterone (a female hormone secreted by the ovary after ovulation) increases risk of endometrial cancer (cancer of the uterine lining) 5- to 14-fold in women who still have their uteri. The addition of progesterone reduces this risk.

2. May increase the risk of breast cancer by 30 percent to 60 percent.[9] These risks are very much disputed.

Advantages of ERT/HRT

1. Reduces loss of calcium from the bones, lowering the risk of osteoporosis
2. Eliminates hot flashes and night sweats
3. Prevents drying and shrinking of vaginal and urinary tract tissues
4. Reduces mood swings

Note that synthetic progestogens and natural progesterone are distinctly different. Natural progesterone is identical to the progesterone produced in a woman's body. Synthetic progestogens are similar but not identical, and more side effects seem to occur with the synthetic progestogens. (See Chapter 32.)

Disadvantages of HRT

1. Although studies are still inconclusive concerning the effects of progestins and heart disease, natural progesterone and nonandrogenic progestins, like Provera, do not raise the blood lipids (fats) as much as androgenic progestins do.[10]
2. May cause bloating, cramping, breast tenderness, nausea, and depression
3. May cause uterine bleeding
4. May increase risk of breast cancer (studies are inconclusive)

ERT/HRT cannot eliminate aging and skin wrinkling. However, estrogen supplementation does make the skin a little plumper and less dry, because of increased collagen production.[11]

Pills, Patches, Injections, and Creams

Pills

Estrogen can be taken by mouth in pill form. It enters the body, is absorbed through the digestive tract, is processed by the liver, and then enters the bloodstream.

Patches

Skin patches allow low, steady doses of the hormone to enter the bloodstream directly, bypassing the liver. This avoids much trouble with liver and gallbladder problems. Although long-term studies are needed to determine the effects on heart disease, osteoporosis, and breast cancer, patches do help with menopausal complaints. However, 20 percent of women will develop rashes from the patches, which are placed on the abdomen or hip twice a week.

Injections

Injection of estrogen directly under the skin allows a slow absorption into the blood without having to go through the stomach or liver first. These injections are usually given by a physician every three to four weeks.

Creams

Vaginal estrogen creams can be applied once or twice a week to help relieve vaginal dryness or urinary problems. When the estrogen dosage is very low, little estrogen enters the bloodstream, lessening both the risks and benefits of estrogen to the body's tissues. However, higher dosages of vaginal estrogens will be absorbed well and have more-pronounced systemic effects.

Progestin creams have also been used to eliminate the

problems associated with menopause and PMS. The application depends on the individual woman and problem. Progestogen therapy is useful in women who cannot take estrogen or who have developed side effects to estrogens.

Androgen cream may be effective in preventing vaginal dryness. Testosterone creams may increase a woman's libido after a hysterectomy. However, there may be permanent masculinizing effects from its use, such as a deepened voice, increased facial hair, and an enlarged clitoris.[12]

Summary

1. The use of ERT/HRT is a very individualized decision. Be aware of the facts and risks before making a decision.
2. ERT protects against cardiac disease (the number one killer of women over age 50). One study suggests that ERT reduces the risk of cardiovascular disease by 40 percent to 60 percent.[13] However, ERT was generally given only to healthy women, which may account for reduced incidences of heart attack with estrogen users.[14] It may increase the risk of breast cancer (the research is contradictory).
3. Studies comparing HRT and cardiac diseases have been fewer than with ERT. Some have conflicting results as to the advantages. HRT may also raise the rate of breast cancer more than ERT.
4. Some women find relief from hot flashes and vaginal and urinary tract problems by taking ERT or HRT for a short time and then discontinuing the treatment gradually.[15] Many women use the treatment for less than one year for menopausal complaints, but most take it for much longer.
5. Women with a uterus should take progesterone along with their estrogen to prevent endometrial cancer.

There is a 5- to 14-fold increase of cancer reported with ERT alone.

6. Both ERT and HRT reduce the risk of osteoporosis by reducing bone loss. The time necessary for using hormones as a preventive for osteoporosis is unknown. Some researchers state that the necessary treatment period may be 6 years, some say 10 years, and some say lifetime treatment. A bone density test can be done to see if you need ERT/HRT for this purpose.
7. ERT is generally recommended for younger women who have had ovariectomies. However, natural progesterone is sometimes supplemented.
8. Apparently the longer a woman is on ERT/HRT, the greater the risk of breast cancer, especially for women who are genetically predisposed.

26
EXERCISE

As women age, fat mass increases and muscle mass decreases. Bone density declines as well. Generally women who have little muscle development also have a subnormal amount of bone.[1] However, the situation is not hopeless: we can all help our bodies by exercising. A study that examined muscle strength and aging found that people up to age 96 were able to increase their muscle size and strength by up to 200 percent.[2] The research shows that for overall good health, specifically of our hearts and bones, both aerobic and weight-bearing exercises are essential. The following are some benefits of exercise:

- Helps to prevent heart disease. Lack of exercise has been established as a risk factor for heart disease. A sedentary lifestyle increases the risk of a heart attack by almost two times.[3] The data from more than 40 studies indicate that coronary artery disease is 1.9 times more likely to occur in inactive people.[4]

- Helps blood vessels transport blood and oxygen to every cell in the body
- Increases bone strength and helps prevent osteoporosis (see Chapter 23)
- Stimulates the ovaries and adrenal glands to produce estrogen
- Improves lung function and increases efficiency of oxygen use in tissues
- Controls weight
- Relieves tension
- Controls high blood pressure
- Can help control cigarette smoking
- Increases energy levels and resistance to fatigue
- Improves ability to sleep
- Increases flexibility

To improve heart and lung condition, activities must raise the heart and breathing rates for periods of at least 30 minutes and must be done no less than three to four times a week. Activities that increase bone strength include weight-bearing exercises and aerobic exercises three times a week.

The American Heart Association states that the following exercises should be done very vigorously for 30 minutes three to four times a week at more than 50 percent of your exercise capacity:[5]

Aerobic dancing
Bicycling
Cross-country skiing
Hiking (uphill)
Ice hockey
Jogging
Jumping rope
Rowing
Running in place
Stair climbing
Stationary cycling
Swimming
Walking briskly

The following activities should be done briskly for 30 minutes or longer three or four times a week:

Downhill skiing	Soccer
Basketball	Squash
Field hockey	Tennis (singles)
Calisthenics	Volleyball
Handball	Walking moderately
Racquetball	

The following activities do not have aerobic benefits but are helpful for muscle tone and strength. They must be done regularly and with exertion.

Badminton	Housework
Baseball	Ping-Pong
Bowling	Shuffleboard
Croquet	Social dancing
Football	Softball
Gardening	Walking leisurely
Golf (on foot or by cart)	

Source: Reproduced with permission. © "Exercise and Your Heart," 1993, copyright American Heart Association.

To be most effective, aerobic activities must be done using the large muscle groups in a rhythmic manner at an intensity that raises the heart rate to 50 percent to 75 percent of its maximum capacity. This ideal heart rate percentage varies with each person and her age.

The information from the American Heart Association that follows gives the maximum heart rate and target rate zone at various ages.

Age (years)	Target Heart Rate Zone (50–75% of maximum in beats/minute)	Average Maximum Heart Rate (100% in beats/minute)
20	100–150	200
25	98–146	195
30	95–142	190
35	93–138	185
40	90–135	180
45	88–131	175
50	85–127	170
55	83–123	165
60	80–120	160
65	78–116	155
70	75–113	150

Source: Reproduced with permission. © "Exercise and Your Heart," 1993, copyright American Heart Association.

During and after exercising, place your first two fingers on your carotid artery, the blood vessels in your neck on either side of the Adam's apple. Or you can check your pulse on the inside of your wrist, just below the thumb. Count the heartbeats for 10 seconds and multiply that number by six. Check your total against the chart. If you are too low, put a little more effort in the exercise. If the number is too high, slow down a bit. When the pulse rate is too high, the effect is anaerobic: the body cannot keep up with the demand for oxygen, and the maximum benefits of exercising cannot be realized. One general rule is that you should always be able to talk and carry on a conversation while you are exercising.

It may be important to check with a doctor before you begin exercising or to help you find an appropriate exercise program, especially if you have a history of heart disease or high blood pressure or are on medication. After choosing the activity, build endurance slowly over a few weeks. Start the exercise with a warm-up period, including stretching. After exercising, end with a cool-down period, also including stretching. Listen to your body. If something causes pain, stop! Check with a physician if you have any pain or pressure in the left- or midchest area, left neck, or left shoulder/arm or if you suffer light-headedness, cold sweats, pallor, or fainting. These may be signs of heart problems.

Kegel Exercises

Women also have a specific need to exercise the pelvic area. These exercises can be made a part of a daily routine. They can be done while doing other exercises, such as abdominal exercises, or even while sitting in the car.

During the late 1940s, Arnold Kegel, a UCLA surgeon, designed a special set of exercises for women who complained of urinary incontinence. Leaking urine can happen gradually throughout the day or as a result of a sneeze, a cough, or laughter. The exercises Dr. Kegel developed proved to be surprisingly effective in restoring bladder control. The exercises focus on strengthening the pubococcygeal muscle, which supports the bladder and the urethra.[6] Properly developed, this muscle can stop the flow of urine in midstream, control bowel movements, and add to increased sexual satisfaction (during sexual activity it contracts rhythmically with orgasm).

Dr. Kegel's first 500 cases had an 84 percent rate of restoration of urinary continence during the exercise program. The study included some women in their 80s who found the exercises effective even though surgery had not corrected their problems.[7]

Learning and performing these exercises are not difficult, but the target muscles must first be identified in order to know what to strengthen. Many adult women do not know how to identify these muscles. One way to accustom yourself to the feeling of contracting the pubococcygeal muscle is to stop the flow of urine when going to the bathroom. Another way is to insert one or two fingers into the vagina and try to squeeze the finger(s) with the inner muscles. Soon you will be able consciously to contract the muscle to exercise and strengthen it.

Described below is the easiest way to learn how to do the exercises. After the technique is learned, it can be done anywhere.

1. Lie on your back on the floor or on a firm surface. It is not necessary to be uncomfortable, so use a mat or rug to rest on.
2. Draw up the pelvic floor, the target muscles, and squeeze. Hold for three seconds and then relax. Repeat this five times.
3. Tighten the muscles slowly up toward the abdomen as high as possible and then slowly release them back down. A number of authors have compared the muscles to an elevator in a building that has five floors. At each elevator stop, hold the muscles tight, count to five, and move up to the next floor. Continue all the way up to the fifth floor, or as high as the muscles will allow, and then relax the muscles at each floor on the way down. Repeat the series five times.
4. Pretend to draw water into and up the vagina. Repeat this five times.[8]

A convenient method incorporates these exercises into an abdominal workout: with every crunch or sit-up, squeeze the target muscles or tighten them, pulling upward toward the abdomen. Using the entire group of muscles at full range seems to be the most effective workout.

Diet and Exercise

Researchers who have looked at the effect of vitamins and minerals on exercising performance have concluded that maintaining an adequate diet is critical to performing one's best and that marginal vitamin and mineral intakes through an inadequate diet result in poor athletic performance.[9] In a review of the subject, another researcher concluded that poor diets, not exercise, are probably the main reason for most mineral deficiencies in athletes; exceptions seem to be iron and zinc, which may well be depleted by heavy exercise.[10] Supplementation may be important for good health, but little evidence exists that it helps athletic performance. On the other hand, numerous studies can point to significant biochemical differences in exercising individuals who take antioxidants such as beta-carotene, vitamin E, and vitamin C. These vitamins do apparently protect against oxidative tissue damage that is otherwise seen during or after heavy exercise.[11] Furthermore, recent data suggest that eating carbohydrates prior to and even ***during*** exercise is beneficial in increasing endurance[12] and reducing the breakdown of muscle protein.

Earlier recommendations for protein intake in athletes have turned out to be probably too low. As much as 5 percent to 6 percent of the calories burned during exercise come from metabolizing muscle tissue. This translates into an increased need for dietary protein during most athletic training.[13]

To date, research has found no magic formulas to enhance exercise performance, but several possibly helpful tips are available:

- Vegetarian athletes need to be especially aware of the difficulties of obtaining protein, iron, zinc, calcium, and vitamin B_{12} from a purely vegetarian diet.[14] They may need to consider broadening their diets or taking supplements.
- Thiamine requirements are dependent on carbohydrate intake. This may be important because some athletes load carbohydrates.[15]
- The requirements of riboflavin are possibly higher in women athletes.[16]

- Vitamin C is thought to improve heat acclimatization in athletes.[17]
- Vitamin E may be helpful when exercising in high altitudes.[18] There is also evidence that supplementation protects against muscle damage during exercise and increases the rate of rebuilding muscle tissue, especially in older individuals.[19]
- Although chromium picolinate has been touted as a natural steroid, we could not find data to back the anecdotal claims. However, chromium is known to significantly influence insulin metabolism and thus may also affect the metabolism of fats and muscle protein. (See Chapter 11.)
- Women athletes tend to be at risk for low iron levels because of low iron intakes and menstrual loss. Long-distance runners, both male and female, are also at risk for low iron levels.[20]
- Magnesium levels have been shown to be low after exercising, but so far no need for supplementation has been established.[21]
- Zinc levels are generally found to be low in athletes, but supplementation has not been shown to affect strenuous activity.[22]

Athletes with low caloric intakes need to eat food high in calcium, zinc, magnesium, B_{12}, and iron. On the other hand, athletes who have high caloric intakes should try to eat foods high in the B vitamins.[23] One authority recommends that the optimal diet for athletes should have the following proportions: 60–75 percent of calories in carbohydrates, 15–20 percent of calories from protein, and no more than 20–30 percent of calories from fats.[24]

The American and Canadian Dietetic Associations currently recommend protein intakes of 1.0 to 1.5 grams per kilogram (g/kg) of body weight for training athletes, as opposed to the recommended daily allowance of 0.8 g/kg.

27

Fish Oils

PRIMARY FUNCTIONS

May reduce risk of heart disease
May reduce risk of atherosclerosis
May reduce blood pressure

Fish oils (omega-3 fatty acids, or n-3 fatty acids) have been purported to reduce, in a number of different ways, the risk of coronary artery disease, in which the coronary arteries are reduced in interior diameter, usually due to atherosclerosis, and blood flow to the heart muscle is decreased. These oils have been shown to lower cholesterol and triglyceride levels, reduce the stickiness of blood platelets, and increase platelet survival. Small amounts of fish in the diet also provide retinol, selenium, vitamin D, and taurine (a compound of unknown function found in high concentration in the brain).[1]

Fish oil has been shown to suppress production of an agent that causes smooth muscle cell growth in the lining of arteries. This may decrease a tendency to form atherosclerotic plaques.[2] Men given fish oil therapy seven days before coronary *angioplasty* (an invasive procedure in which a blocked or injured artery is dilated/repaired) and for six months following have shown less than one-half the rate of reblockage than controls did.[3] Restenosis (reblockage) of the coronary arteries after angioplasty is a major problem, often requiring repeat angioplasty or a bypass operation.

Another study looked at men and women with large-artery atherosclerosis. The subjects' diets were supplemented with low doses of omega-3 fatty acids (4 teaspoons of cod-liver oil per day). The results indicated that they had prolonged platelet survival times by more than 20 percent. This likely represents a decrease in clotting tendency, which may translate into a decreased chance of heart attack.[4]

Researchers have suggested that some polyunsaturated fats can lower blood pressure. One study, conducted to determine the effects of n-3 polyunsaturated fats (fish oil) and n-6 polyunsaturated fats (safflower oil) on blood pressure, administered different combinations of the fats to men with mild essential hypertension (high blood pressure with no discernable cause). The results of the study indicated that high levels of fish oils are effective, whereas safflower oil is not. However, the researchers were concerned about the safety of high doses of fish oils.[5] A later review indicated that fish oils may be most helpful in persons with hypertension, atherosclerosis, or high cholesterol but showed little effect on the blood pressure of normal individuals.[6]

Fish oils are known to lower levels of plasma triglycerides but have been shown variously to raise, lower, or have no significant effect on cholesterol levels. These diverse effects may depend on whether the fish oils are replacing or just supplementing animal fats in the diet.[7]

Greenland Eskimos' very low death rate from coronary heart disease has been ascribed to their diets being high in fish. Studies have compared the effects of diets both rich and poor in fish consumption. One sampled 852 middle-aged Dutch men who began the study without heart disease. In a 20-year follow-up, 78 men had died from heart disease. A 50 percent reduction of mortality due to heart disease occurred in the men who consumed at least 30 grams (g) of fish a day. The researchers concluded that eating fish one to two times a week may have a preventive value against heart disease.[8]

No specific recommended daily allowance (RDA) has been given. The above-mentioned study supports eating fish one to two times a week. However, a supplemental capsule of fish oil is available. It is sold as EPA (eicosapentaenoic acid), generally in doses of 200 or 500 milligrams (mg).

Liver and fish liver oils contain large amounts of vitamin A, which may cause toxicity (see Chapter 3). High intakes of fish oils may increase lipid peroxidation in tissues. The increased need for concomitant antioxidants such as vitamin E to counter this effect is unknown at this time.[9]

28

FOOD

Poor diet contributes to many diseases. It has been shown to promote cancer, coronary heart disease, osteoporosis, stroke, obesity, and diabetes mellitus. A good diet, on the other hand, is one of the major foundations of good health.

Many different health and governmental organizations have recommendations for a "good" diet. Generally, these guidelines are very similar. They all agree on the importance of maintaining a healthy body weight, eating a wide variety of foods from all the major food groups, and imbibing no more than one to two drinks of alcohol per day. Most recommendations include a reduction of fats to less than 30 percent of the total calories consumed. Less than 10 percent of dietary fats should be saturated fats. Most organizations agree on the need for an increase in both fiber and carbohydrate foods. Cholesterol intake should be no greater than 250 to 300 milligrams (mg) per day. Their recommendations vary on sodium; most say sodium consumption should be less than 3 grams (g) per day.

Guidelines

The guidelines presented here are from different health and government agencies. Their similarities become obvious after perusal of the list.

American Institute for Cancer Research*

- Reduce the intake of dietary fat—both saturated and unsaturated—from the current average of approximately 37 percent to a level of 30 percent of total calories, and reduce the intake of saturated fat to less than 10 percent of total calories.
- Increase the consumption of fruits, vegetables, and whole-grain cereals.
- Consume salt-cured, salt-pickled, and smoked foods only in moderation.
- Drink alcoholic beverages only in moderation, if at all.

FDA Consumer[1]

Amounts per day:

Calcium	800 mg (women 25 and older)
Iron	15 mg
Calories	2,200 (women 23-50) to maintain weight; don't cut back to less than 1,500 when dieting
Cholesterol	Not more than 300 mg
Fat	Not more than 30 percent of total calories, with less than 10 percent from saturated fats

**Menus and Recipes to Lower Cancer Risk* (Washington, D.C.: American Institute for Cancer Research, 1991). Reprinted with permission from the American Institute for Cancer Research.

U.S. Departments of Agriculture and Health and Human Services[2]

Servings per day:
Vegetables, 3–5
Fruits, 2–4
Breads, cereals, rice, and pasta, 6–11
Milk, yogurt, and cheese, 2–3
Meat, poultry, fish, dried beans, peas, eggs, and nuts, 2–3

American Heart Association*

- Total fat intake should be less than 30 percent of calories.
- Saturated fatty acid intake should be less than 10 percent of calories.
- Polyunsaturated fatty acid intake should be no more than 10 percent of calories.
- Monounsaturated fatty acids should make up the rest of total fat intake, about 10 to 15 percent of total calories.
- Cholesterol intake should be no more than 300 milligrams per day.
- Sodium intake should be no more than 3,000 milligrams (3 grams) per day.
- Eat no more than 6 ounces (cooked) per day of lean meat, fish, and skinless poultry.
- Try main dishes featuring pasta, rice, beans, and/or vegetables. Or create "low-meat" dishes by mixing these foods with small amounts of lean meat, poultry, or fish.

- The approximate 5 to 8 teaspoon servings of fats and oils per day may be used for cooking and baking, and in salad dressings and spreads.
- Use cooking methods that require little or no fat—boil, broil, bake, roast, poach, steam, saute, stir-fry, or microwave.
- Trim off the fat you can see before cooking the meat and poultry. Drain off all fat after browning. Chill soups and stews after cooking so you can remove the hardened fat from the top.
- The three to four egg yolks per week included in your eating plan may be used alone or in cooking and baking (including store-bought products).
- Limit your use of organ meats such as liver, brains, chitterlings, kidney, heart, gizzard, sweetbreads, and pork maws.
- Choose skim or 1% fat milk and nonfat or low-fat yogurt and cheeses.

To round out the rest of your eating plan:

- Eat five or more servings of fruits or vegetables per day.
- Eat six or more servings of breads, cereals, or grains per day.

American Cancer Society[3]

- Maintain desirable weight. Individuals 40 percent or more overweight increase their risk of colon, breast, prostate, gallbladder, ovary, and uterus cancers. Physicians can recommend a suitable diet and exercise regimen to help maintain an appropriate weight.
- Eat a varied diet. A varied diet eaten in moderation offers the best hope for lowering the risk of cancer.

- Include a variety of vegetables and fruits in the daily diet. Studies have shown that daily consumption of vegetables and fruits is associated with a decreased risk of lung, prostate, bladder, esophagus, and stomach cancers.
- Eat more high-fiber foods such as whole-grain cereals, breads, and pasta; vegetables; and fruits. High-fiber diets may reduce risk of colon cancer. Such diets offer a healthy substitute for fatty foods.
- Cut down on total fat intake. A diet high in fat may be a factor in the development of certain cancers, particularly breast, colon, and prostate.
- Limit the consumption of alcohol, if you drink at all. The heavy use of alcohol, especially when accompanied by cigarette smoking or smokeless tobacco use, increases risk of cancers of the mouth, larynx, throat, esophagus, and liver.
- Limit consumption of salt-cured, smoked, and nitrite-cured foods. In areas of the world where salt-cured and smoked foods are eaten frequently, there is more incidence of cancer of the esophagus and stomach. The American food industry has developed new processes to avoid possible cancer-causing by-products.

U.S. Department of Health and Human Services[4]

- Choose foods high in dietary fiber daily (fruits, vegetables, and whole-grain breads and cereals).
- Choose foods low in dietary fat.
- If you drink alcoholic beverages, do so only in moderation.
- Avoid unnecessary x-rays.
- Health and safety rules of your workplace should be known and followed.

- Avoid too much sunlight: wear protective clothing; use effective sunscreens.
- Take estrogens only as long as necessary.
- Above all, don't smoke! Tobacco causes about one-third of all cancer deaths—more than all the other reliably known cancer-causing agents added together. Heart disease and emphysema caused by smoking kill even more people than does cancer.

U.S. Departments of Agriculture and Health and Human Services[5]

1. Eat a variety of foods. No one food provides all the nutrients that a person needs. It is important to eat a wide variety of foods each day, such as fruits and vegetables; whole cereals; lean meats, poultry without skin, and fish; dry peas and beans; and low-fat dairy products.
2. Maintain healthy weight. Obesity is a risk factor for many diseases, including heart disease, high blood pressure, diabetes, and some cancers.
3. Choose a diet low in fat, saturated fat, and cholesterol. A diet low in total fat may reduce the risk for cancers of the breast, prostate, colon, and rectum. Such a diet will probably be low in saturated fat and cholesterol and may also reduce the risk of heart disease.
4. Choose a diet with plenty of vegetables, fruits, and grain products. Most Americans eat a diet low in starch and fiber. Health experts recommend that we increase the amount of starch and fiber in our diets by eating more fruits, vegetables, potatoes, whole-grain breads and cereals, and dry peas and beans. A high-fiber diet may reduce the risk of colon and rectal cancer.

5. Use sugars only in moderation. A diet high in sugar promotes tooth decay. Sugary foods are often also high in fat and calories and low in vitamins and minerals.
6. Use salt and sodium only in moderation. Too much salt in the diet may contribute to high blood pressure, especially for people with a family history of high blood pressure. Untreated high blood pressure can lead to heart attacks, strokes, and kidney disease.
7. If you drink alcoholic beverages, do so in moderation. Drinking too much can lead to many health problems. Heavy drinking is associated with cancers of the mouth, throat, esophagus, and liver. Cancer risk is especially high for heavy drinkers who smoke. Alcoholic drinks are also high in calories and low in vitamins and minerals.

American Heart Association*

Blood (serum) Cholesterol milligrams/deciliter	*Classification*
Less than 200 mg/dl	Desirable
200–239 mg/dl	Borderline high
240 mg/dl and over	High

Low-density Lipoprotein (LDL) Cholesterol	*Classification*
Below 130 mg/dl	Ideal
Between 130 and 160 mg/dl	Borderline high risk
Over 160 mg/dl	High risk

*Reproduced with permission. © *Cholesterol and Your Heart*, 1991, 1993, copyright American Heart Association.

Forty percent of Americans have blood cholesterol levels greater than 200 mg/dl, which doubles their risk for coronary heart disease compared to those with much lower cholesterol levels.[6]

Protein

Total protein intake should not be more than 15 percent of the total calories consumed. The recommended dietary allowance (RDA) for a woman over age 25 is 0.8 grams per kilogram of body weight. Depending on a woman's weight, protein intake should be approximately 30 to 70 g per day. This daily protein requirement can be satisfied by eating two eggs or 4 ounces of meat or chicken and a glass of milk.[7] One gram of protein is equal to 4 calories. High-protein diets have been associated with increased loss of calcium in the urine, which can be detrimental to bone density. Animal protein sources are generally high in fats, which have been associated with heart disease, cancer, and weight gain.[8]

Amino Acids

Twenty amino acids are known to be the building blocks of human protein. Nine of these cannot be synthesized by the body and therefore must be assimilated from the diet; these are known as essential amino acids. The others are called nonessential amino acids since the body can manufacture them from other compounds. The intake of essential amino acids needs to be balanced, or protein synthesis will be hampered.

Protein can be termed complete or incomplete. Complete protein contains eight of the nine essential amino acids. The ninth, *histidine*, is thought to be essential for infants and children but probably not for adults. Arginine, often classed as nonessential, can be arguably placed in the essential group since the body's ability to synthesize it cannot keep up with needs during growth. Incomplete protein lacks essential amino acids, therefore requiring other food sources to complete it. Complete protein foods are seafood, poultry, meat, eggs, cheese, and milk. Incomplete protein foods include grains, legumes, and other vegetables.

It is beyond the scope of this book to explore the research on amino acids. However, they are ingredients in many of the nutritional supplements on the market. As with vitamins and minerals, claims are made that we get all of our amino acid nutrients from an average diet, and claims are made to the contrary.

AMINO ACIDS

Essential	*Nonessential*
Histidine	Alanine
Isoleucine	Arginine
Leucine	Asparagine
Lysine	Aspartic acid
Methionine	Cysteine
Phenylalanine	Glutamic acid
Threonine	Glutamine
Tryptophan	Glycine
Valine	Proline
	Serine
	Tyrosine

SUGAR

Sugars are simple carbohydrates that offer no vitamins or minerals. One gram of sugar is equal to 4 calories. Common sugars are either monosaccharides or disaccharides; that is, they are made up of one basic sugar unit or two units linked together. The monosaccharides are glucose (dextrose), fructose, and galactose. Disaccharides are combinations of these in double units.

Sucrose, from sugar beets and sugar cane, is plain table sugar. It is a disaccharide composed of the monosaccharides fructose and glucose, both found in fruits and honey. Fructose is also made commercially from cornstarch. Other disaccharides are lactose and maltose. Lactose is milk sugar. Maltose is malt sugar, used in the fermentation of beer, produced in breadmaking, and found in legumes.

The average person in the United States consumes about 125 pounds of sugar per year. This is equivalent to approximately 18 percent of total calories consumed. Consuming the average of 2 pounds of sugar per week represents 3,600 calories, the equivalent of almost 1 pound of fat. Reducing sugars is a helpful way to reduce weight gain.[9] Unwanted weight gain results from eating too many calories regardless of the source. Cutting back on added sugar is a good way to cut calories without reducing nutrients. Also, too much sugar can lead to tooth decay and can also predispose postmenopausal women to vaginitis by raising the vaginal pH, inviting infection.[10]

Complex Carbohydrates

Complex carbohydrates (starches and dietary fiber) are long strands of simple sugars. Many health agencies recommend that at least half the calories consumed be from carbohydrates. Carbohydrates have been linked to a reduction in the risks of colon cancer and heart disease. They are found in grains, peas, beans, fruits, potatoes, and vegetables. One gram of carbohydrate is equal to 4 calories.

Starches

Starches, such as potatoes and pastas, are good food sources for energy. Starches by themselves are not high in calories; it is all the fatty and high-calorie stuff people put on them that makes them fattening.[11]

Fiber

Fiber is the nondigestible parts of plants. It also consists of complex carbohydrates made up of long chains of simple sugars. But the sugars are linked differently than they are in starch, and our digestive enzymes can't break them down. Diets high in fiber may help prevent digestive disorders, hemorrhoids, and cancer of the colon and rectum, help with weight management, and lower serum cholesterol levels.[12] The National Cancer Institute recommends 20 to 30 g of fiber per day. Fiber can be either soluble or insoluble. Soluble fiber is found in beans, fruits, oat bran, vegetables, and brown rice. It may help lower blood cholesterol levels. Insoluble fiber is found in whole-grain products and again in fruits and vegetables. It helps provide bulk necessary for the formation of stools.

Diets high in fiber may inhibit the absorption of some minerals and vitamins. Women who eat high-fiber diets may have an increased need for both calcium and magnesium.[13]

Fats

Fats are a necessary part of the diet. They are needed among other things for energy, for cell membrane structure, and to transport fat-soluble nutrients such as vitamins A, D, E, and K throughout the body. Most health agencies recommend that less than 30 percent of total calories come from fats and less than 10 percent from saturated fats. One gram of fat is equal to 9 calories, so the above recommendation translates into 65 g of fat in a 2,000-calorie diet. Fats occur in several different forms:[14]

Cholesterol

A fat-like substance, *cholesterol* is both manufactured by the body and consumed in the diet. It is needed to make bile salts, hormones, and vitamin D. High cholesterol levels have been associated with increased risk of heart disease. Cholesterol is found in animal products, dairy products, fish, and shellfish.

Triglycerides

Triglycerides are fats made up of three fatty acids attached to a glycerol molecule. In the body these are the major transport and storage form for fats. High levels of triglycerides have been associated with heart disease and diabetes.

Unsaturated Fats

Monounsaturated fats, found primarily in olive, canola, and peanut oil, may help to lower cholesterol levels. *Polyunsaturated fats* are mostly vegetable oils that are liquid at room temperature. Some are omega-6 fatty acid–containing oils such as soybean, safflower, corn, sunflower, sesame, and cottonseed. Also in this group are the omega-3 fish oils (see Chapter 27), which have been shown to lower blood cholesterol levels.

Saturated Fats

Saturated fats are generally found in animal products and some vegetable oils. They are usually solid at room temperature. Saturated fats are known to raise cholesterol levels in the blood. They are found in meats, dairy products, some fatty fish, coconut oil, palm oil, palm kernel oil, whipped toppings, and nondairy coffee creamers.

Trans-Fatty Acids

In the United States, daily per capita animal fat consumption decreased from 104 g in 1909 to 97 g in 1972, while the consumption of vegetable fats increased from 21 g to 59 g. Thus animal fats decreased from 83 percent to 62 percent as a proportion of Americans' total fat intake during a period of time that authorities were diligently warning us about the dangers of animal fats predisposing to heart disease and cancer.[15] But while the consumption of animal fats was falling, heart disease and cancer rates were rising. Something didn't make sense. That something may well be *trans*-fatty acids.

As early as the 1950s, researchers posed a concern over processed vegetable fats and their effect on health. A process called hydrogenation is used to transform unsaturated vegetable oils such as soybean oil into less saturated oils and fats. This accomplishes two things. It gives them a longer shelf life, with less tendency to become rancid. Also, it can convert oils into fats, that is, oils that are solid at room temperature. The latter can be used for margarines, spreads, and shortenings. Today partially hydrogenated vegetable shortenings have largely replaced lard, butter, and other animal fats in the U.S. baking industry. However, synthetic hydrogenation produces *trans-fatty acids*, chemically altered unsaturated fatty acids that have a different type of carbon-carbon double bond than is found in naturally occurring fats. According to estimates, the daily per capita intake of *trans*-fatty acids rose from 4.4 g in 1910 to 12.1 g in 1972.[16]

Unfortunately it has taken about 30 years for these concerns to be given serious attention, but recently the literature has more and more studies critical of *trans*-fatty acids. These fats have been shown to raise low-density lipoprotein (LDL) cholesterol and to lower high-density lipoproteins (HDLs);[17] they alter immune response, change cell membrane structure, and perhaps most ominously alter some enzyme systems that metabolize carcinogens and drugs.[18] Indeed, some investigators have found associations between *trans*-fatty acids and increased risk of heart disease in women, as well as breast cancer.[19] Expect to hear more unfavorable news about *trans*-fatty acids and hydrogenated fats and oils over the next few years.

Try to eat monounsaturated fats in favor of other fats and limit the use of polyunsaturated fats, especially hydrogenated vegetable oils. Cookies, donuts, deep-fried foods, chips, imitation cheese, and pastries that are not made with butter or lard are full of *trans*-fatty acids from partially hydrogenated oils;[20] so are margarines and spreads. In general, the softer the item, the less hydrogenation. For example, liquid or tub margarine has less hydrogenation than stick margarine.[21]

Sodium

As the body ages, kidney function slows down, and the body is less able to rid itself of excess sodium. Too much sodium in the diet may increase the risk of high blood pressure, kidney failure, and heart disease. Many health agencies recommend that we eat less than 3 g of sodium per day. The average person in the United States consumes about 4 to 6 g of sodium per day. Our bodies require only 0.5 g of salt or 0.2 g of sodium per day. Generally 30 percent of salt intake comes from the use of salt at the table and in food preparation, and 70 percent is derived from that naturally present in foods and from commercial processing of foods. Other sources of sodium are listed below.[22] Reducing sodium intake is one of the first reasonable approaches in hypertensive women.[23]

SODIUM SOURCES

Baking soda	Baking powder
Monosodium glutamate	Sodium caseinate
Sodium saccharin	Sodium benzoate
Disodium phosphate	Sodium nitrate
Sodium citrate	Some sleeping aids
Some antacids	

Water

A woman's body is composed of about 60 percent water. Water helps carry nutrients, hormones, and oxygen throughout the body. It also is responsible for flushing out waste products. According to recommendations, a woman should drink six 8-ounce glasses of water per day.[24]

Alcohol

The jury is still out on the effects of alcohol. Some say that longevity is increased in moderate drinkers. Alcohol does have an overall positive effect of raising HDL_3 (a subfraction of HDL), but whether this provides any protection against coronary heart disease is disputed. It also has been shown to increase blood pressure and impair glucose tolerance. It depletes vitamin A, thiamine, riboflavin, biotin, choline, B_6, folic acid, niacin, calcium, and magnesium.[25] Some of the effects of drinking alcohol are insomnia, liver damage, depression, increased susceptibility to infection, inhibition of the immune system, and increased risk of high blood pressure and cancer. It also promotes hot flashes during the climacteric (menopause, or "change of life").[26]

Caffeine

Caffeine (found in coffee, tea, and colas) constricts the blood vessels, elevates body temperature, causes high blood pressure, and can trigger hot flashes. Excess caffeine consumption depletes vitamin C, calcium, zinc, potassium, and the B vitamins.[27]

The tannins in coffee and tea reduce the absorption of many minerals, especially iron. It has been suggested that less than two cups of coffee a day will not have any negative health risks.[28]

29
The Female Heart

Breast cancer and osteoporosis have received top billing as women's health issues because they are "women's diseases." But cardiovascular disease, a supposedly male problem, is *the* major cause of death in women over 50 years old. Approximately 247,000 women in the United States die each year from heart attacks, whereas 28,000 women die of breast cancer and fewer than 2 percent of women older than 65 will die from osteoporosis-related hip fractures.[1] A woman is twice as likely to die in the two weeks following a heart attack than is a man. One in seven women between the ages of 45 and 64 has some form of heart disease. This rate increases to one in three after the age of 65.[2] Coronary heart disease is 1.9 times as likely to occur in inactive people as in people who exercise. More than half the people living in the United States have blood cholesterol levels greater than 200 milligrams/deciliter, which puts them at risk for coronary heart disease. Most studies on exercise and heart disease have been conducted on young and middle-aged men; studies on women and girls are limited, and results of the studies are inconclusive.[3]

The Heart

The normal heart is a muscle that acts as a pump, moving approximately 2,000 gallons of blood a day. The heart beats, filling and contracting, about 100,000 times a day. It consists of four chambers; the top two are called *atria*, and the bottom two are called *ventricles*. Blood is pumped through them in an organized and systematic fashion. Four valves control the one-way directional flow of blood. The right side of the heart is a relatively low-pressure system, pumping blood from the body to the lungs; the left side is a high pressure system, pumping blood from the lungs to the body.

First the right atrium fills with blood, which has traveled throughout the body and has returned to the heart via the veins. This blood is highly saturated with carbon dioxide and carries little available oxygen. When the atria contract, blood flows into the right ventricle. Next the ventricles contract, which pushes the blood into the pulmonary artery and on to the lungs. As blood passes through the lungs, the carbon dioxide in the blood diffuses into the *alveoli* (small, bubblelike sacs in the lungs) and is expelled. At the same time, in the other direction, oxygen diffuses across the alveolar membranes and is picked up by hemoglobin, the oxygen-carrying, iron-containing proteins in red blood cells. Thus replenished, the oxygenated blood flows into the left atrium and then into the left ventricle. With another ventricular contraction, the oxygenated blood is pushed through the aorta, the body's major artery, and distributed throughout the entire circulatory system.

The circulatory system is a network of elastic tubing that takes oxygen and nutrients to all parts of the body. This system also picks up the body's waste products and delivers them to the liver, lungs, and kidneys, where they are filtered, excreted, exchanged, or metabolized.

Diet and the Heart

Diet has been shown to be a major player in the development of heart disease, and reduction of fat and salt intake is urged. As is widely known, excess salt consumption is one of the common contributors to high blood pressure, which in turn contributes to heart disease. More fascinating, however, is the recent concern over *trans*-fatty acids, commonly found in partially hydrogenated vegetable fats and oils. It turns out that the rise in heart disease in the United States more closely follows the increase in use of these oils than it does the consumption of animal fats, which has actually declined since 1900.[4] For more on *trans*-fatty acids and for the American Heart Association's dietary guidelines, refer to "Guidelines" and "*Trans*-Fatty Acids" in Chapter 28.

30

HERBS

For centuries, plants around the world have been used for medicinal purposes. Generally, in the United States, plants have been replaced by synthetic products. However, there seems to be a reawakening of interest in the use of plants for health and medicinal purposes. This is demonstrated by the number of fast-growing herbal companies that have opened their doors in the last few years.

There is little room to doubt that many plants have medicinal value. Yet their administration and use carry inherent problems. To begin with, determining dosage is very difficult, as is controlling quality in a plant. The concentration, or potency, of the constituents in each plant is determined by the soil, location, climate, season, and other uncontrollable factors. Second, the plant often contains nonbeneficial or even harmful substances that ideally should be avoided. Third, the optimal durations of herbal therapies are unknown. Fourth, little information is available on the short- and long-term side effects of various herbs. And last, most of the information available on herbal therapy comes from anecdotal testimonies and folklore, not rigorous scientific research. Few scientific studies have been done, most of them animal based.

These are not problems limited to "radical" herbal medicine. Until a few years ago, many of the above statements could have been made (and were) about one of the most widely used heart drugs in the world—digitalis, an extract of foxglove. Debate continued for years over the advantages of various extracted components versus pills made from the whole leaf. One of the major problems with both treatment and research was the inability to standardize dosage, since the potency of the product varied greatly according to source, growing conditions of the foxglove, and so on. Two lessons learned from the "herbal research" on digitalis and heart disease were that dosage standardization is difficult and that too much of a wonderful thing can be extremely poisonous.

The present discussion will be limited to garlic, onions, some plants producing estrogenic effects, and a few herbs commonly used for some female problems. Garlic is actually recognized by the Japanese food and drug authorities as a treatment for hypertension. Both garlic and onions have been researched for their value in reducing blood cholesterol and cancer risk. Soybeans have been researched for their value in inhibiting the growth of certain cancers and their role in lowering the risk of breast cancer. Still other plants produce chemical compounds that exhibit estrogenic activity in both humans and animals; these chemicals are called *phytoestrogens* (i.e., plant estrogens). This group of plants includes soybeans, yams, apples, barley, carrots, winter cherry, coffee, green beans, oats, parsley, peas, pomegranate, potatoes, red beans, rape, rice, rye, sesame, wheat, yeast, ginseng, licorice, fennel, unicorn root, false unicorn root, alfalfa, red clover, dong quai, sage, and black cohosh.[1] In addition, phytoestrogens have been identified in beer (containing hops) and bourbon (made from corn).[2]

Garlic

In a review of the genus *Allium*, both garlic and onion were shown to be effective inhibitors of platelet aggregation (essential for clotting) in human blood. They were also shown to prevent increases of plasma fibrinogen (the inactive form of fibrin, a major blood-clotting protein) and reductions in blood coagulation time and fibrinolytic activity. In plain English, this means that garlic and onion may help lower the risk of blood clots and thereby reduce the risk of strokes. Onion and garlic have also been shown to reduce serum cholesterol and triglycerides.[3] In Germany, Kwai (a Chinese garlic) is licensed as a drug for the treatment of atherosclerosis; in the United States it is considered a dietary supplement.[4] People who eat as little as 10 grams (g), or ⅓ ounce (oz) per week of garlic and 200 g (6–7 oz) per week of onion were better protected than people who abstain. However, those who eat 50 g (almost 2 oz) per week of garlic and 600 g (20 oz) per week of onion show even greater benefits.[5] A very recent review of placebo-controlled, randomized studies ascertained that high-cholesterol patients could reduce their cholesterol levels by an average of 9 percent by eating as little as one-half to one clove (not bulb) of garlic daily.[6]

In a double-blind, placebo-controlled study, subjects who took 800 milligrams (mg) per day of garlic powder over a four-week period had significant beneficial changes in their blood: inhibited blood clot development, increased circulation in capillaries (the networks of tiny blood vessels throughout the body), and decreased blood sugar values.

These blood changes quite possibly could have an effect on reducing the risk of heart disease and helping patients with diabetes.[7]

Garlic consumption was shown to be strongly associated with low risk of colon cancer in a 1994 study, with a 35 percent reduction of risk among garlic eaters. This was a more striking association than was found with any other fruits, vegetables, or dietary fiber studied in a group of over 40,000 women.[8] Epidemiological studies in China have shown that the dietary intake of garlic is inversely related to the incidence of gastric cancer.[9]

Fresh garlic also has been shown to be effective as an antibacterial agent against both Gram-positive and Gram-negative organisms, even against some organism strains that have become resistant to common antibiotics. The compound allicin is the active antibacterial agent in garlic, and its use or that of synthetic analogs as antibacterial agents is worth further exploration.[10]

Phytoestrogens

Phytoestrogens were first studied in the 1920s. To date, approximately 300 different plants are known to produce these compounds, which are about $\frac{1}{400}$th as potent as estradiol in the human body.[11] Phytoestrogens are not actually estrogens, but they can bind to estrogen receptors and elicit a similar response.[12] Tamoxifen, a popular drug that is widely used to treat breast cancer, has a structure similar to some phytoestrogens.[13]

Estrogen receptors are very complex and not well understood. The phytoestrogenic agents are thought to work in the following manner: The body has a limited number of estrogen receptors, which can be occupied by either estrogen or phytoestrogen or can be vacant. If the majority are bound by estrogen, then the estrogenic activity is high. If the majority are vacant, then the estrogenic activity is low. Introduction of phytoestrogens moderates the above situation. In low-estrogen states, phytoestrogens will increase estrogenic activity by binding to empty sites. In high-estrogen states, they will reduce estrogenic activity by displacing some of the estrogen molecules with less potent substitutes. Michael Murray and Joseph Pizzorno, the authors of *Encyclopedia of Natural Medicine*, add that, as opposed to estrogen, phytoestrogens have not been associated with an increased risk of cancer.[14]

Researchers, while agreeing that phytoestrogens simulate the effects of estrogen, argue about their practical value for treatment of specific problems. An additional problem is that most of the available data are based on animal studies. Interpreting the results from animal studies and extrapolating them to humans may have limited validity. For example, some animals tend to develop pancreatic enlargement and liver disease when consuming diets high in phytoestrogens, whereas this has not generally been found true in humans.

Soybeans are probably the most thoroughly researched of the phytoestrogen-producing plants. The phytoestrogens in soybeans belong to a chemical family called isoflavones. Soybeans also contain a few different anticarcinogens and growth inhibitors, which have been shown to inhibit or prevent the development of experimentally induced colon, lung, liver, oral, and esophageal cancers in animals.[15] A recent study of Japanese men and women who ate a traditional Japanese diet concluded that the low incidence of breast and prostate cancer among the Japanese may be linked to their high intake of soybeans.[16]

Some interesting effects from phytoestrogens have been recorded. According to Hopkins et al., uterine bleeding in a postmenopausal woman was caused by the use of a Chinese ginseng face cream; the phytoestrogens absorbed through her skin had been enough to influence her uterine lining.[17]

In animals, sterility problems have been attributed to the consumption of phytoestrogens. Sterility has been reported in Australian sheep grazing on subterranean clover, a phytoestrogen-producing plant.[18] Infertility and liver disease are common problems seen in captive cheetahs fed diets high in soy protein. Researchers concluded that soy isoflavones in the diet are likely responsible.[19] A contraceptive effect was noted in a study on rabbits and rats fed castor plant (*Ricinus communis* var. *minor*) seeds;[20] these results were also found in a study on rats given injections of extracts of winter cherry fruit, a traditional contraceptive recommended by Iranian herbalists. The rats had a 96 percent reduction of pups, and their progesterone levels decreased by 44 percent. When the treatments stopped, the pregnancy rate increased to normal levels.[21]

Until recently, yams were a major source of medicinal estrogen products. They were eventually replaced with synthetic and animal estrogens. Premarin®, a conjugated estrogen, is derived from *pre*gnant *mar*e's ur*in*e, an abundant and inexpensive source of estrogen.[22]

Herbs Commonly Used for Female Disorders

Recently there has been an explosion of preformulated vitamin, mineral, and herbal remedies available from retail stores, mail-order houses, and multilevel marketing businesses. A close reading of the labels will often find one or more of the following herbs in the preparation. Brief descriptions explain the rationale for their inclusion in the group. WARNING: All contraindications that apply to estrogen use also apply to the use of herbs with phytoestrogens (see Chapter 25). Not enough data are available at this time to recommend the use of these herbs without warning.

Phytoestrogen Herbs

Dong Quai Dong quai roots have been used for most gynecological complaints, including premenstrual syndrome (PMS), irregular menstrual flow, abdominal pain, and lack of vaginal lubrication.

Ginseng There are three major types of ginseng: Siberian (*Eleuthrococcus senticosus*); American (*Panax quinquefolium*); and Chinese (*Panax ginseng*). *Panax ginseng* is the most widely used. The roots seem to increase activity of the adrenal glands and are touted to increase sexual endurance. Estrogen-like effects were seen in the vaginal lining of a postmenopausal woman taking *Panax ginseng* for a two-week period.[23] WARNING: Ginseng has been reported to raise blood pressure, but these claims are hotly disputed.

Sage Sage has been used to regulate menstrual flow and relieve hot flashes.

Black Cohosh The roots and rhizomes of black cohosh supposedly relieve cramps associated with menstruation and reduce hot flashes and excessive bleeding. The herb has been administered during childbirth to reduce pain and stimulate uterine contractions. WARNING: Large doses can cause nausea and dizziness.

Licorice Root Licorice roots are used for aiding digestion, treating upper respiratory problems, and relieving stress. Licorice works as a muscle relaxant, stimulates mucus production, and exhibits antiviral properties. WARNING: Licorice can raise blood pressure and can cause water retention and loss of potassium.

Fennel and Anise Both fennel and anise have been used to increase milk production, produce menstruation, facilitate birth, alleviate hot flashes, and increase libido. Toxicity problems are rare. In 1970 the Council of Europe proposed no restrictions on fennel oil use. The U.S. Food and Drug Administration has approved it for food use.[24]

Nonphytoestrogen Herbs

Red Raspberries The leaves, bark, and roots of red raspberries are used for PMS and menstrual cramps. The herb helps to decrease menstrual blood flow. WARNING: Red raspberry leaves may inhibit the absorption of iron.

Goldenseal The roots and rhizomes of goldenseal are used for just about everything. Goldenseal purportedly boosts the immune system, and almost every organ and disease state has been claimed to benefit from its effects. WARNING: Do not use for long periods of time. It can cause stomach problems.

Damiana Damiana leaves help relieve headaches and increase intestinal contractions. It is touted in Mexico as an aphrodisiac. WARNING: Damiana is known to interfere with iron absorption.

Sarsaparilla The roots of sarsaparilla are used for regulation of hormones.

31

Menopause

Natural *menopause* has technically arrived when menstruation has ceased for one year. Surgical menopause occurs abruptly at the time of surgery, when ovaries are removed. The *climacteric* is that period of years during which the body uses the last of its eggs and hormonal changes begin to occur. As the number of eggs decreases, the levels of estrogen and progesterone produced by the ovaries begin to fluctuate. The pituitary no longer perceives the higher, premenopausal levels of hormones and works harder to promote them. In its attempt to stimulate the ovaries to release eggs, the pituitary raises the follicle-stimulating hormone (FSH) as much as 13 times and raises the luteinizing hormone (LH) levels 3 times. Eventually, without ovulation, estrogen levels drop, progesterone production ceases, the uterine lining does not thicken, and menstruation stops. After menopause has occurred, estrogen is made from androstenedione, a weak male hormone produced in the ovaries and adrenal glands and converted into estrogen by fat, liver, and kidney tissues.[1]

Menstruation may end very gradually, abruptly, or erratically. In the United States 10 percent of women go through menopause by the age of 38, 30 percent by the age of 44, 50 percent by the age of 49, 90 percent by the age of 54, and 100 percent by the age of 58. Women who are thin, smoke cigarettes, have had twins, have had less education, and have lower incomes tend to experience menopause earlier than other women.[2]

With menopause many women experience hot flashes, headaches, sleeplessness, mood swings, vertigo, heart palpitations, shortness of breath, asthma, fatigue, libido changes, and digestive problems. Internally the vagina can change from being moist and reddish in color to dry and pale. The cervix changes from being soft to firm. The breasts may change: smaller breasts tend to become smaller and flatter; larger breasts tend to elongate and droop; nipples become smaller and may lose their ability to become erect.[3] The bladder and urethra (urine canal) lose muscle tone and decrease their production of fluids that help to ward off infection.[4] (See Chapter 33.) Unfelt initially but eventually more important are losses in bone mass that may lead to osteoporosis.

The good news is that birth control problems are solved, and women who suffered with premenstrual syndrome (PMS) find that problem alleviated. Women who stop menstruating abruptly either naturally or surgically tend to have more problems than women who go through the hormonal changes gradually. Also, thin women tend to have more acute problems than heavier women. Sudden drops in estrogen level or low estrogen reserves accompanying low body fat appear to amplify the discomforts.

Every woman experiences the "change of life" differently. Up to 10 percent to 15 percent of women slide through these years not noticing any difficulties, and 10 percent to 15 percent are severely debilitated.[5] However, the majority of women have at least a few bothersome problems.

Hot flashes occur in up to 85 percent of women and are very troublesome for 10 percent to 20 percent. They can disrupt sleep night after night, leaving a woman exhausted and worn down. When a hot flash occurs, the skin temperature rises 4–8 degrees Fahrenheit, and the body temperature drops.[6] They generally occur for about 2 years, 20 percent last for 5 years, and in a small number of cases they can persist up to 10 years or more.

When the levels of estrogen drop, the mucous membranes, skin, and urogenital tissues are affected. The skin loses its moisture, and the vaginal mucosa (membrane) can become thin and dry, resulting in painful intercourse. There also can be a thinning and drying of the urethral tissues, causing painful urination and problems with incontinence.

Some women find that they have an increased libido (sexual desire), some notice a decrease, and some notice no change at all. Androgens are major contributors that can affect sexual interest and desire. During the climacteric and postmenopausally there is a drop in estrogen levels but a plateau in testosterone levels. Some researchers have attributed elevated libido to higher testosterone levels. Decreased libido can occur in women who have had ovariectomies, or removal of the ovaries, because the ovaries produce androgen as well as estrogen. However, we women are not totally ruled by our hormones. A woman's feelings about sex, herself, her partner, and the world around her strongly influence her interest and desire for sex.[7]

With the thinning, shrinking, and drying of the vagina, sexual activity may be less comfortable. It may take longer to produce enough fluids for penetration; lubricants may be necessary. Also, sexual sensation may be less pronounced due to decreased blood flow to the vaginal area.

Mood swings may also be produced by the drops and fluctuations of estrogen and progesterone levels. Lowered estrogen levels also are known to cause sleep disturbances.

The following treatments have been used for menopausal problems (see Chapter 35, "Recommendations"):

- Hormone replacement therapy (HRT—for women with a uterus) and estrogen therapy (ERT—for women without a uterus) relieve many of the problems associated with midlife and menopausal complaints. ERT and HRT have been shown to reduce or completely stop hot flashes, reduce bone loss, and possibly reduce the risk of heart disease. However, these therapies have side effects. They are not for everybody. (See Chapter 25.)
- Vaginal lubricants such as K-Y jelly, vegetable oil, saliva, and massage oils can be helpful for vaginal dryness.
- Estrogen cream may also be helpful in relieving vaginal dryness. (See Chapter 25.)
- Testosterone creams have been said to increase a woman's libido. However, these may have masculinizing effects. (See Chapter 25.)
- STOP SMOKING! Smoking makes hot flashes more severe;[8] increases your risk of heart disease, cancer, osteoporosis, and lung disease; and shortens your life span.
- Start exercising or continue to exercise. Exercise may help to lessen severity of hot flashes. It also reduces the risk of heart disease and osteoporosis and reduces stress that may be associated with hormonal changes. (See Chapter 26.)
- Vitamin E has been used for relieving hot flashes. Some people have suggested taking 1,000 international units (IU) per day of vitamin E, either with or without 500 milligrams (mg) of vitamin C, and 25 micrograms (mcg) of selenium. Check with a physician if you have high blood pressure or are taking digitalis. (See Chapter 3 and Chapter 7.)

- Vitamin A supplementation has been used for vaginal dryness.
- Other herbs such as dong quai and licorice root have been used to relieve hot flashes and vaginal dryness. (See Chapter 30.)
- Clonidine, a blood pressure medication, has also been used to relieve hot flashes. Check with a physician.
- Do not let your body fat drop below 15 percent. This reduces the amount of estrogen in your body. A little fat is in and will help a little with estrogen production.
- Feed your bones. Many physicians and researchers recommend that you supplement your diet with 1,000 mg of calcium premenopausally and 1,500 mg postmenopausally. However, more aggressive authorities would advocate 1,500 mg and 2,000 mg, respectively. Include in your supplement vitamin K, magnesium, manganese, boron, phosphorus, and zinc.
- Take care of your heart. Try to eat more vegetables and fruits high in beta-carotene; more polyunsaturated fats, fish, soybeans, and whole grains; and less meat. Postmenopausally reduce your iron intake and eliminate it from supplementation. Check with your physician. (See Chapter 29.)

Read *Silent Passages* by Gail Sheehy, *Natural Menopause* by Susan Perry and Katherine O'Hanlan, *No More Hot Flashes* by Penny Wise Budoff, M.D., and *The Pause* by Lonnie Barbach. They are wonderfully written, informative books on the topic of menopause.

32

Premenstrual Syndrome (PMS)

Premenstrual syndrome (PMS) has a wide range of symptoms that recur monthly. The syndrome has been attributed to a disorder in the endocrine system, but the exact cause of the syndrome is unknown, as is the remedy. Although no cure has been found for PMS, there are recommendations to reduce many of the symptoms. General remedies include limiting certain foods and eating others, vitamin and mineral supplementation, exercise, and reduction of stress. Some medical treatments include hormonal and psychoactive agents.

Ruling out other medical disorders such as hypoglycemia (low blood sugar), thyroid problems, and manic depression is important. Each of these disorders presents many of the same symptoms as PMS. In the case of hypoglycemia it is important to have the blood sugar levels drawn during the premenstruum, which are the days immediately preceding menstruation.[1]

Foods that should be avoided are sugar, processed foods,

refined carbohydrates, caffeine, alcohol, and salt. The foods suggested as helpful include complex carbohydrates, fruits, and vegetables. Also advisable is eating many small meals per day rather than a few larger ones and drinking plenty of water. However, be sure to maintain the total caloric intake. Exercise is essential to alleviate stress and enhance general health.

Although supplementation with B_6 (pyridoxine) has been used as a treatment for PMS, its value has been disputed. In one study on premenstrual anxiety, irritability, and nervous tension, the symptoms of PMS were reduced when the women received 200 to 800 milligrams (mg) per day of B_6. The women in this study had high levels of estrogen and low levels of progesterone; 200 to 800 mg of B_6 reduced the estrogen levels and increased the progesterone levels. Also, according to the report, B_6 reduced water retention problems by lowering levels of aldosterone (a kidney-regulating hormone).[2] In another double-blind, placebo study, similar results were found. Of 25 women with PMS receiving 500 mg of B_6 per day for a three-month period, 21 experienced fewer symptoms of PMS.[3] However, chronic vitamin B_6 supplementation has been shown to be toxic at low doses. In one study, over 100 women taking an average of 117 mg of B_6 per day for six months to five years reported neurological symptoms. When the supplementation of B_6 was stopped, the women completely recovered from their symptoms within six months.[4]

Lethargy and muscle weakness occurring throughout the cycle may be attributed to a depletion of potassium, especially if diuretics have been used. During the premenstrual period, sodium and water are retained in the body, and potassium is reduced through urination. Potassium supplementation or extra servings of fruits and vegetables, but not juices, may be helpful to relieve these symptoms.[5] (See Chapter 20.)

According to reports, many of the most common complaints of PMS may be attributed to magnesium deficiency. Magnesium deficiency causes a drop in brain dopamine levels without a commensurate drop in norepinephrine or serotonin, causing anxiety and depressive symptoms.[6] (Dopamine, norepinephrine, and serotonin are all nerve messenger chemicals in the brain.) Also, chocolate cravings may be an indication of a magnesium deficiency.[7] A magnesium to calcium ratio of 2 to 1 has been suggested for relief of many PMS symptoms.[8] However, the generally accepted magnesium to calcium ratio is approximately 1 to almost 3. The magnesium/calcium balance is critical to preserving bone density. (See Chapters 10, 16, and 23.)

One treatment for PMS is natural progesterone. (Natural progesterone and synthetic progestogens are not equivalent agents; the synthetic progestogens do not have exactly the same effects on the body as natural progesterone does, and they generally result in more side effects.)[9] Natural progesterone treatments may be administered by injection, pill, or suppository. The female hormone has been shown to beneficially affect most PMS symptoms except restlessness and decreased sexual arousal.[10] The use of natural progesterone therapy has been an accepted treatment for PMS in Britain for many years. No major side effects have been noted over a 30-year period with the use of the therapy.[11]

Another common treatment for PMS is estradiol. Both estradiol implants and transdermal (administered by applying a patch to the skin) estradiol suppress ovulation. It is not known if the reduction of PMS symptoms is due to the disruption of the menstrual cycle or due to suppression of ovulation. However, as opposed to naturally occurring estradiol, *conjugated estrogens* (such as Premarin) have been shown to exacerbate the symptoms.[12]

Other hormonal treatments include danazol, leuprolide, and oral contraceptives. Although these are purported to relieve the symptoms of PMS, they are not free of side effects.[13] Another often prescribed treatment, tranquilizers, can be effective but may easily lead to abuse. Antidepressants are prescribed for acute levels of depression. Check with your physician. There are new medications available all the time. An excellent review of the treatments available for PMS is the article "Pharmacologic Strategies for Managing Premenstrual Syndrome," by Margaret L. Moline (see the Bibliography). It is well worth reading by anyone with more than passing interest in the subject.

33

SKIN AND AGING

The skin performs a number of functions critical to health and well-being. The *epidermis* (the outside layer of the skin) prevents fluid loss and protects the lower levels of skin from physical insults of the outside world as well as from microorganisms. With the help of melanin (skin pigment), it protects against the carcinogenic effects of ultraviolet radiation. The *dermis* (the inner layer of the skin) controls body temperature by increasing or decreasing the blood flow through the skin's circulatory system and by regulating the activity of the sweat glands. The *subcutis* (subcutaneous fat, the bottom layer of the skin) serves as padding to protect the organs beneath, as well as providing insulation and energy storage. The total weight of all bodily skin on an adult has been estimated at 7–9 pounds, with an area of 20 square feet. It is the largest organ of the body.[1]

Epidermis: The Outer Layer of Skin

The epidermis contains several layers of cells: the stratum corneum—a dead, horny, surface layer made up largely of the protein keratin—and the deeper layers of live cells. These are the granular, spinous, and basal cell layers. The layers of skin vary in thickness, depending on location. For example, the epidermis is very thick on the palms and soles but is very thin in the vagina and on the eyelids. The epidermis develops from the basal cells on its deep aspect. The basal cell layer, by cell division, produces a constant supply of new skin cells. These mature into flat, tough, keratin-filled, platelike cells that form the horny, dry skin surface. The outer layer is continuously sloughed off, leaving newer skin cells showing. The entire growth of the skin from the basal layer to the epidermal surface takes approximately one month. If this process is not interrupted by any extraneous influences, it will produce smooth and pliable skin.

Two functional rather than structural cell types are found in the epidermis: the melanocyte and the Langerhans cell. *Melanocytes* derive from the same embryonic tissue that gives rise to brain and nerves. However, these specialized cells produce a pigment called ***melanin***, which gives all of us our distinct skin and hair colors. These are variations of yellow, brown, and red. Our own genetic makeup determines what our skin and hair colors will be. Melanin is an excellent absorber of ultraviolet light. The denser the melanin, the darker the skin color and the more built-in protection from the sun.

The Langerhans cells are derived from the bone marrow and play a role in the skin's immunology. These cells can capture and process antigenic materials (substances capable of triggering an immune response) that come in contact with the skin and can eliminate them through the lymphatic system. Langerhans cells are decisive in determining immunity, tolerance, or allergy to various substances.

Dermis: The Lower Skin

The dermis is also thick or thin depending on the specific region of the body. For example, the dermis is very thick on the back but very thin on the palms. This lower skin layer is made up of collagen and elastin set in a web of jellylike matrix (glycosaminoglycans). The elastin fibers, intertwined with the collagen, are the main reason why skin is elastic. The glycosaminoglycans act like a sponge holding water. This material controls how much moisture our skin contains. Within the collagen-elastin network is a maze of blood vessels, nerves, sweat glands, ducts, and lymphatics (vessels that contain or convey lymph). The nerve sensors enable us to feel touch, pressure, temperature, and pain. Oil glands, or sebaceous glands, which are largest and most numerous on the face, chest, scalp, and back, produce many different fats and waxes. This mixture of fats and waxes, called *sebum*, is secreted from the oil gland into a duct or hair follicle and moves from there to the skin surface. Sebum lubricates the skin and protects it from drying out.

Pores are the openings to sweat and oil glands located in lower skin layers. The size of the pores is mostly determined by heredity and age.

The Subcutis

The subcutis, a subcutaneous fat layer, protects the organs beneath and is a storage area for energy and nutrients. The quantity of fat cells is thought to be largely determined by heredity. This layer houses the apocrine glands and the eccrine glands. *Apocrine glands* are usually found in the armpits and breast areolae (skin around nipple), around the belly button, and in the genital and anal regions. They produce milky sweat that is secreted into the upper section of the hair follicle and eliminated to the skin surface. This secretion is attacked by bacteria and causes body odor. The *eccrine glands* are common sweat glands. They have ducts to transport sweat directly to the surface. Sweat consists of water and a few salts, is odorless, and is produced in response to exercise, heat, stress, and fevers. It cools the body by evaporation.

Aging Skin

Many of the skin changes that happen in our 30s, 40s, and 50s are wrongly blamed on menopause. Most of these changes, wrinkles (our character lines) and spots, are due to aging, heredity, cigarette smoking, sun damage, and other environmental factors. When we are young, the skin growth cycle may take as little time as two weeks. However, between the third and seventh decade there is a 50 percent decrease in the cell turnover rate.[2]

Prior to significant sun exposure, the skin in young children has a very orderly geometric pattern. The epidermis has a network of infolding ridges that reach down into the dermis. These form a geography of plateaus and crisscrossing valleys at the interface of the dermis and epidermis, resulting in an increase in surface area at that interface. In aged skin, the overall geometry remains the same, but the entire epidermis is thinner, decreasing approximately 20 percent in thickness over one's lifetime.[3] The rete (network) ridges disappear and diminish the area of contact between the dermis and the epidermis. The valleys are shallower and the plateaus are larger. The epidermal turnover rate is decreased by 30 percent to 50 percent. This results in slower skin growth, a possible reason why older folks don't heal as well as younger ones. Both the melanocytes and the Langerhans cells appear decreased in number as people age, and the pores tend to become larger. Presently no products are on the market that really will shrink the pores for more than a few hours.[4]

In the skin of a small child, the fine collagen bundles are in a very simple pattern parallel to the skin's surface. In older skin, the collagen bundles are tightly packed and randomly oriented. Collagen is thought to decrease up to 1 percent a year during adult life.[5] Whether there is a gradual or rapid loss of glycosaminoglycans is in dispute. One theory suggests a loss of glycosaminoglycans and a flattening of collagen resulting in the filling of empty spaces and crowding of elastin fibers.[6] Consequently, there is thinning of the dermal layer and a loss of resiliency of the skin and its ability to retain water. Elastin fibers decrease in number, unravel, fragment, and straighten, which results in a loss of elasticity.[7] A decrease in circulation and in the function of the sweat glands also occurs. Women have an estimated 32 percent reduction per decade in sebum (oil) production after the age of 20.[8] As a result, our skin becomes drier as all of us age.

Premature Aging: Sun Damage

Skin exposed to the sun one too many times has distinctly different physical characteristics than nonexposed skin. Women who have had a life of sun exposure look older than women who have had little sun exposure.[9] The most obvious effects are increased wrinkling, uneven pigmentation, and increased risk of cancer.

The skin first loses its geometric pattern, which may result in cracking and fissuring.[10] The melanin in our skin acts as a sunscreen, but through years of exposure to the sun the pigment cells become damaged and lose their protective ability. Melanocytes are two to three times as numerous in exposed skin as in nonexposed skin.[11] The increase in the number and density of the groupings of the melanocytes alternating with areas of loss creates "age spots" and uneven tanning. A loss of pigment cells through the natural aging process only compounds the problem for future sun exposure. This melanocyte loss and damage leaves us less protected, adding to the direct assault of the ultraviolet rays on our skin. In the dermal layer, the collagen fibers have a decreased resiliency, and the elastin fibers turn into shapeless, fuzzy clumps.[12] These changes leave a blotchy, cancer-prone skin with a leathery, nonelastic texture.

Skin Cancer

In the United States more than 600,000 cases of basal cell and squamous cell skin cancers are diagnosed yearly. Almost all of these cases are thought to be related to sun exposure. Fortunately both cancers have a very high cure rate. Melanomas are strongly suspected to be related to solar radiation.[13] There were 15,000 cases reported in women in 1992; an estimated 2,600 women in the United States will die this year from melanomas. More cases of skin cancer are reported near the equator, and people with lighter skin color are more susceptible.[14]

Smoking

Tobacco smoking damages collagen and impairs the blood circulation to the skin. Constriction of blood vessels results in a decrease in nutrients and oxygen delivered to the various layers of skin. The result is yellowish skin color, crosshatched wrinkles on the face, a lot of tiny and not so tiny lines all around the mouth, and crow's-feet by the eyes. Cigarette smoking is also estimated to be responsible for 79 percent of lung cancer in women and for 30 percent of all cancer deaths.[15]

Heat, Cold, and Weight Loss

People exposed to extreme temperatures in their environment or in the sauna are more likely to wrinkle. The temperature extremes put extra stress on the skin. People who lose weight may have a problem with cutaneous elasticity, causing extra wrinkles and saggy skin. Sometimes skin is not resilient enough to follow the new shape of the body.[16]

"Spots and Things"— and What to Do About Them

Seborrheic Keratoses

Seborrheic keratoses are harmless, hard, or scaly black, brown, or grey spots on the skin. They are often velvety, rough, or warty. They may be removed by liquid nitrogen, electrodesiccation (dehydration using a high-frequency electrical current), or surgery. One must remember that, depending on the site, size, and removal technique, treatment may leave a scar that is more noticeable than the spot.

Actinic Keratoses

Actinic keratoses, caused by chronic sun exposure, are rough, scaly, and usually pinkish or reddish-brown. They are precancerous and should be treated. Depending on the location, size, and thickness, treatment may involve liquid nitrogen, electrodesiccation, acid application, dermabrasion (using an abrasive to plane, or "sand," the skin), curettage (cutting away), or treatment with a chemotherapy cream.

Basal Cell Carcinomas

Basal cell carcinomas are very common raised, bumpy, or flat spots that may bleed, scale, and sometimes be confused with pimples. Basal cell skin cancers need to be treated. Although they can cause extensive local destruction if not treated when small, they have no significant tendency to metastasize (spread to other organs).

Squamous Cell Carcinomas

Another common form of skin cancer, squamous cell carcinomas are bumpy, scaly, crusted, or warty pinkish growths that tend to bleed and become inflamed. These may metastasize throughout the body, although it is uncommon.

Malignant Melanomas

The most serious and least common of the major skin cancers are malignant melanomas. They may resemble moles, may be flat or raised, but usually have irregular or indistinct borders. As they develop, their color may change to include blue, black, red, tan, white, and brown. Any new or recently changed mole or pigmented spot is suspect. Any spot with multiple colors or irregular color distribution is suspect. Any spot or mole with irregular borders is suspect. Treatment is simple and curative if the cancer is diagnosed early, but the cancer is often fatal if detected late.

Spider Veins (Telangiectases)

The tiny veins that mostly appear on the legs or cheeks are nothing more than prominent superficial (near the skin surface) capillaries. They supply neither nutrition nor oxygen to the areas. Spider veins may be removed for cosmetic reasons by electrodesiccation, sclerotherapy (injection of a caustic solution, such as strong saline, which destroys the vessel), or laser treatments.

Cherry Spots (Cherry Angiomas, Senile Angiomas)

Cherry spots are usually small, raised, red spots that appear on the skin more and more frequently with age. They are harmless but may be bothersome cosmetically or physically, depending on location. They are quite easy to remove with liquid nitrogen or electrodesiccation.

Skin Tags

Skin tags are small, harmless extra flaps of skin that may be annoying. Women over 40 and postmenopausal women are prone to growing them. There is also a familial predisposition. They usually appear around the neck, eyelids, groins, armpits, and shoulders. These can be removed by electrosurgery, excision, or liquid nitrogen.

Moles (Nevi)

Generally, moles are harmless. They can be flat or raised and are usually brown, tan, or pink. However, they should be watched carefully for any irregularity or changes in size, color, texture, or border shape, as well as any tendency toward bleeding or inflammation. These signals may herald a change into a melanoma (cancer) and need to be checked by a dermatologist.

Cysts

Sebaceous glands in the dermis sometimes form a sac filled with a harmless cheese-like substance. Usually, a large pore leads to the skin surface. So-called sebaceous cysts are frequently found on the back, scalp, or face and range in size from a small bean to a Ping-Pong ball. On the head they are commonly called *wens* and often cause bald spots on the overlying scalp due to chronic pressure impeding blood flow to the hair follicles. Occasionally the cysts become inflamed and swell up like boils. Cysts can be removed surgically if inflamed or uncomfortable or for cosmetic reasons.

Age, or Liver, Spots (Senile Lentigines)

It might be preferable to call age spots by their literal translation: "freckles of old age." Changes in pigmentation due to clustering of melanocytes, they are large dark spots and are harmless. Bleaching creams will reduce the color over a few months, but the spots will return if the area is exposed to the sun. Liquid nitrogen, chemical formulas, cryotherapy (using extreme cold), and electrosurgery are used to remove the spots. Once again, scarring or white spots may be more noticeable than the initial lesion.

Sun Damage Prevention, Treatments, and Procedures

Treatments and skin care products are available that will rejuvenate some damaged skin, but the best course is to avoid sun damage to begin with. All of us will have some wrinkles eventually, but healthy and attractive skin is possible despite them.

Use a good sunscreen with a sun protection factor (SPF) of 15. Sunscreens with SPFs of 30 or above may actually cause dryness problems due to the higher concentrations of chemicals in the sunscreen. Presently many good sunscreens are available. There are gels and creams for the sports-minded or those who perspire heavily; these agents will persist for hours unless you use soap. There are sunscreens for use under your makeup, in your makeup, and as moisturizers. There are sunscreens with para-aminobenzoic acid (PABA) and without. (As many as 5 percent of people get allergies to PABA.) It is a good idea, whether or not you use makeup, to get in the habit of applying some form of a sunscreen in the morning as a protective shield. Just protecting it from the sun will allow your skin to heal itself to some degree and will also deter further damage. If you really want to have a tan, try some of the new skin-staining products. Chemical based rather than radiation based, they will allow your skin to have a darker color.

It has been suggested that sun damage may be mitigated by supplementing the diet with 400 international units (IU) of vitamin E as d-alpha tocopherol acetate and 100 micrograms (mcg) of selenium. For immediate relief, taking approximately 2,000 IU of vitamin E along with one or two aspirins will help alleviate a sunburn and its inflammation. The vitamin E must be taken soon after the sun exposure.[17] But in light of other reports that the damage done by radiation may depend on the total antioxidant pool in the body, balancing all of the antioxidant vitamins is probably the most prudent course.

Whether or not you use sunscreens or take antioxidants, wear clothes that will protect you from the sun, including dark polarized sunglasses, a wide-brimmed hat, and long sleeves.

Tretinoin, known as Retin-A®,[18] is a vitamin A derivative. This drug has received a tremendous amount of attention since 1988. It was almost exclusively used to treat acne before it was reported to rejuvenate sun-damaged skin. It makes the skin more youthful looking by removing the top layers of dead skin scales, plumping out fine wrinkles, and fading much of the blotchy, brown pigmentation that accompanies sun-caused aging (photoaging). In addition, Retin-A appears to repair some of the damage done to the skin's blood vessels and to incite production of new, healthy collagen over old, sun-damaged collagen. Side effects may include skin irritation and an increased susceptibility to sunburn, windburn, and winter chapping. The U.S. Food and Drug Administration has not yet approved the use of Retin-A for wrinkles.

Two new drugs on the market, Vivida[19] and Imedeen,[20]

are both treatments for sun-damaged skin that are derived from the cartilage of marine fish. European studies have purported to show that treated skin is thicker, has a smoother appearance, and appears to have greater elasticity. The only side effects reported were pimples in the first few weeks of use. Brittleness of both hair and nails was also reported to improve with treatment.[21]

Acid peels are commonly employed procedures for rejuvenating facial skin. They can generally be divided into three classes: light, medium, and deep. As with most things, you get what you pay for. In the case of acid peels, the payment is an increase in risk and pain for deeper peels in return for the promise of more dramatic rejuvenating changes.

Light peels affect only the epidermis. The dermis remains unscathed. This means that only superficial blemishes confined to the epidermis can be treated, including keratoses, many pigmentation problems, and dull, dry skin texture. Wrinkles and scars are not affected by light peels. The advantage is that they are very safe because the dermis is not injured. A variety of agents are used, including Retin-A, trichloroacetic acid, and the new alpha-hydroxy acids such as glycolic acid. Light peels may or may not result in redness and peeling, depending on the agent used. Recovery, however, is quick, at most only a few days. And in general, no time need be lost from your general routine.

Medium-depth peels wound the epidermis and the uppermost dermis. This means that some minor wrinkles can be eradicated, in addition to resurfacing the epidermis. In general, the same agents are used as in light peels but at greater concentrations or for longer exposure times. The recovery times are also consequently longer, and rawness or sheetlike shedding of the facial skin is the rule.

Deep peels wound the dermis relatively deeply. The epidermis is obliterated. Controlled healing results in reorganization of the skin collagen similar to remolding plastic after melting it. Numerous agents are used, but the gold standard of deep peels is the phenol peel. Expertly used, the deep peel is capable of effacing even moderately deep lines and wrinkles and is often used to get rid of the radiating furrows that develop around the mouth. Scarring is a hazard, as is the loss of natural skin pigment in the treated areas, sometimes leaving the patient with a ghostly appearance unless makeup is worn. Cardiac monitoring is routinely done with phenol peels because of the reported heart toxicity of phenol. Recovery is prolonged, and sun avoidance for 6 to 12 months is often required to prevent pigment blotching.

Dermabrasion is a technique that uses high-speed rotating wire brushes or diamond fraises to literally sand your wrinkles away. This procedure may produce scarring, mottled pigmentation, and uneven healing of the skin, just as deep peels do. This also must be performed by a physician.

Collagen injections are used to fill in wrinkles and scars by injecting a creamy preparation of purified cow collagen into the dermis. This is a temporary treatment, because the bovine collagen is gradually metabolized by the body. Touch-up injections must be done every few months to maintain any cosmetic improvement. Allergies to the injected materials may result.

Liposuction is the process of removing fat from subcutaneous areas to change a specific contour of the body.

Microlipoinjection (fat transplantation) is the technique of removing fat, usually from the abdomen, thighs, or buttocks, and using it to fill in scars or wrinkles. The fat is extracted with a large-bore needle, rinsed of blood, and reinjected into the target site. This temporary treatment has the best success if used in places where little skin movement takes place.[22]

Blepharoplasties (eyelid tucks) and facial rhytidectomies (face-lifts) are techniques used to surgically remove sagging and wrinkles.

Nails

The nail consists of dead, cornified (converted into horny tissue) cells that are produced by the nail matrix. The matrix, or nail bud, is located under the cuticle and extends a short distance out under the nail. The only visible area of the matrix is the *lunula*, the whitish moon that can be seen in your nail. The nail itself, properly called the nail plate, is made of many layers of tightly bonded platelets of nonliving substance produced by the matrix. Most of the substance in the nail is keratin, the same protein that makes up skin surface and hair. Much of the flexibility of nails is dependent upon the water content of the nail. This hydration is in turn dependent on the relative humidity. The growth of nails increases in the 20s and 30s and appears to decrease after that as people age. Fingernails grow about 0.1 to 0.25 inch a month, and toenails grow about half as fast. Nails grow faster in the summer months than in the winter or in colder climates. With age may come irregularity of nail growth.[23] Ridges and uneven growth patterns occur. However, most complaints heard from 40- to 60-year-old women are of brittle nails. Such a change may occur suddenly around or some time after menopause. When this happens, the nails remain brittle for about four years and then improve. There does not seem to be any treatment that helps to relieve this problem but time.[24]

Hair

Hair, like the skin's stratum corneum, is mostly a nonliving keratin protein. The hair shaft is located deep in the dermis. The root, at the base of the hair follicle, is the only living and growing part of the hair. Each hair is made up of two parts, the cortex and the cuticle. The cortex is the center support layer, and the cuticle is the outer protective layer. The hair grows in three cycles: the growing (anagen) phase, the involutional (catagen) phase, and the resting (telogen) phase. Approximately 85 percent of the time is spent in the growing phase, 11 percent in the resting phase, and the remaining 4 percent in the involutional or transitional phase.

A woman has an average of approximately 125,000 strands of hair on her head and loses between 50 and 100 hairs a day. There is more hair loss in the late fall, less in the spring. When a hair falls out, the same hair follicle is used to grow a new hair. Actually, when a hair falls out under normal circumstances, it does so because it is being pushed out by a newly growing replacement hair. Generally, scalp hair grows about one-half to three-fourths inch a month. Genetic factors determine hair type, quantity, pattern, and location.

Hair and Aging

During middle age, most women's hair thins and turns gray or white. Very few women lose all their hair; generally thinning is most prominent at the crown, and hair also becomes thinner and finer in the temporal area. Again, the amount of loss is usually dependent on heredity. However, health factors, such as stress and illness, and reactions to certain drugs, notably beta-blockers, can cause hair loss. Also, with aging, the pigment cells disappear from the hair follicle. The number of the melanocytes begins to diminish at about age 30. Gray hair is the result of having only a few melanocytes in the hair follicle, and white hair results from an absence of melanocytes. Gray hair is very strong; it is also more resistant to permanents and dyes. Gray hair tends to have thicker strands and can look beautiful and full.

Hirsutism (Excessive Hair Growth)

When the estrogen level drops and becomes erratic, the balance between estrogen and androgen is disrupted. This may cause the growth of new, thick, coarse, dark hairs—usually in unwanted areas of the body. A couple of medical disorders can also cause the problem, so if more than a few "wild hairs" appear, it might be best to consult a physician.

Vaginal and Urinary Tracts

The vagina is a very adaptable part of the body. It can elongate, stretch, and lubricate itself for sexual activity. It also has the ability to accommodate the birth of a child and then return to its original shape.

In early adulthood the vagina is quite acidic, which helps prevent infection. As women age and approach menopause, less estrogen is produced, causing a decrease in production of vaginal fluids and an alkaline shift in the vaginal pH. The vaginal entrance becomes smaller, the vaginal epidermis becomes thinner and less elastic, and the self-lubricating ability of the vagina diminishes. These changes may result in more-frequent vaginal infections and in discomfort or pain during sexual intercourse.

Also, the bladder and the urethra begin to lose muscle tone over time. The physical changes in the urethra, bladder, and vagina can leave the urethra more exposed to trauma from sexual activity. Combined with a reduction of fluids, these changes increase the risk of bladder infection and inflammation. Incontinence is another common problem associated with the loss of muscle tone. Loss of urinary control can be trivial to extreme. Often this problem is exacerbated by the onset of menopause and a drop in estrogen. Kegel exercises have been used successfully for years to improve bladder control (see Chapter 26). Medications are also used to relieve the problem.

Vaginitis actually comprises a number of disorders, but they all cause an inflammation of the vagina with burning, itching, soreness, and a sometimes odorous discharge. Different factors contribute to vaginitis: antibiotics, douches, deodorants, nylon underwear and pantyhose, wet bathing suits, bath oils and bubble baths, tight pants, intercourse with inadequate lubrication, and intercourse with an infected partner.

As women age, some have more difficulties than others. Some experience very little discomfort, whereas others are miserable. However, almost all women encounter problems to some degree or another. They would be wise to talk to their physicians about solutions, especially when some of the more embarrassing problems, such as incontinence, occur. Always see a physician if problems persist. Many infections and physical discomforts may be signs of other, more serious problems.

You are not alone. After all, this is the generation of the baby boomers. It has been estimated that close to 19 million women next year alone will enter menopause.

Miscellaneous Skin Nutrients and Treatments

- Vitamin C: It has been recommended by some dermatologists to promote healthy skin. Quite a bit of evidence exists that C speeds up wound healing. (See Chapter 5.)
- Vitamin E: Along with vitamin C, this is a major antioxidant and preventer of inflammation and tissue injury. (See Chapter 7.)
- Vitamin A: This vitamin is associated with the development of healthy mucous membranes. (See Chapter 3.)
- Aloe vera: There is some evidence that aloe vera can help alleviate radiation dermatitis. It also promotes healing in chronic leg ulcers, pressure sores, frostbite, and surgical

wounds. Unfortunately, few controlled studies have been done with humans.[25]

- Biotin: This promotes healthy hair and skin. (See "Biotin" in Chapter 4.)
- Calcium: The skin has a calcium-dependent antioxidant enzyme. It has been suggested that a calcium deficiency can accelerate skin aging. (See Chapter 10.)
- Copper: Copper is involved with the production of elastin, collagen, and melanin. (See Chapter 12.)
- Zinc: Zinc has been reported to increase the speed of wound and ulcer healing. (See Chapter 22.)
- Retin-A: This popular drug has been shown to improve photoaged skin.[26] Researchers are not actually sure why the medication works. However, improvements have been noted in fine wrinkling, elasticity, and skin color.

34

WEIGHT

As previously mentioned, lean body mass, or muscle mass, decreases as we age. The percentage of fat goes up, and the amount of muscle goes down. Every year from our middle 30s on, the body requires fewer and fewer calories per day to maintain the same weight. The number of calories necessary to maintain weight declines by an estimated 2 percent to 8 percent per decade.[1]

Ideal body weight is not that which is glamorized by the media or preferred by couturiers. It is a matter of health, not fashion, and it can easily be computed or looked up in appropriate charts (see the chart at the end of this chapter). Women who are 15 percent below the average weight have higher risks of pneumonia, influenza (the *real* flu), digestive-system disorders, ischemic heart disease, and death.[2] This may be due to decreased energy intake rather than to low weight per se.[3] Obese women (30 percent or more over ideal body weight)[4] increase their risk of diabetes, high blood pressure, and death.[5]

Reprinted here is the 1983 Metropolitan Life Insurance Company height and weight table for women aged 25–59, based on the lowest mortality. The weight is measured in pounds according to frame size, including 3 pounds of clothing and 1-inch heels.

WOMEN AGED 25-59

Height in Feet and Inches	Small Frame	Medium Frame	Large Frame
4′ 10″	102–111	109–121	118–131
4′ 11″	103–113	111–123	120–134
5′ 0″	104–115	113–126	122–137
5′ 1″	106–118	115–129	125–140
5′ 2″	108–121	118–132	128–143
5′ 3″	111–124	121–135	131–147
5′ 4″	114–127	124–138	134–151
5′ 5″	117–130	127–141	137–155
5′ 6″	120–133	130–144	140–159
5′ 7″	123–136	133–147	143–163
5′ 8″	126–139	136–150	146–167
5′ 9″	129–142	139–153	149–170
5′ 10″	132–145	142–156	152–173
5′ 11″	135–148	145–159	155–176
6′ 0″	138–151	148–162	158–179

Source: Reprinted courtesy of Metropolitan Life Insurance Company

The relationship between weight and mortality can be viewed as a U-shaped curve. The top of one end of the curve represents the very heavy people and the top of the other end represents the very thin people. Both of these extremes have high mortality rates. This pattern also holds for the hospitalization rate.[6] One 12-year study comparing mortality and body weight reviewed over 17,000 healthy, nonsmoking Finnish women between the ages of 25 and 79. The researchers found that thin and obese women between the ages of 25 and 64 had the highest mortality. However, this pattern of mortality did not hold for women over 64.[7]

Many studies show that the above-mentioned mortality and body weight curves may be true for middle-aged people but not for older people: people 60 and older tend to have a higher mortality associated with thinness than those under that age.[8] Older people appear to require more weight for a given height than younger people do.

Obese people who maintain their weight have lower mortality than do those whose weights fluctuate. A modest, 10 percent or less, weight reduction over an eighteen-month period should be the desired goal. After that goal has been achieved, another reduction can be considered. This modest reduction also appears to have the greatest overall health benefits.[9] One study on weight gain and cardiovascular health followed, over a 10-year period, almost 12,000 Harvard alumni with a mean age of 58. Originally the men were free of cardiovascular disease. Based on the men's responses to questionnaires, the study concluded that significant body weight *gain or loss* was associated with a higher rate of mortality from coronary heart disease and other noncancer causes.[10]

A recent survey found that about 40 percent of adult women are trying to lose weight at any one time. The bad news is that it hardly ever works.[11] Be careful of yo-yo dieting; cyclically losing and regaining weight has been thought to be very detrimental to overall health. And to top it off, the weight lost is usually back within two years. When an individual loses 20 quick pounds, that weight loss represents 5 pounds of muscle and 15 pounds of fat. With resumption of a normal diet, the body, now adjusted to starvation metabolism, has lower caloric needs. Because the body requires fewer calories to maintain weight, when the 20 pounds are regained, 18 pounds are fat and 2 pounds are muscle.[12] This was the gospel according to the weight-loss authority, but just recently the National Task Force on the Prevention and Treatment of Obesity has published a report critical of the yo-yo diet studies. While the task force does not endorse yo-yo dieting, its findings indicate that the fear of regaining weight should not discourage obese persons from trying to shed pounds.[13]

Ideal body weight can be quickly and easily estimated using the Hamwai formula for women:[14]

1. Start with 100 pounds for the first five feet of height.
2. Add five pounds for each additional inch.
3. For a small frame, subtract 10 percent from the total; for a large frame, add 10 percent.

IV
Putting It All Together

35

RECOMMENDATIONS

VITAMIN AND MINERAL DOSAGE RANGE TABLE

Key

The following notes refer to the table beginning on page 214.

1. Column 1 identifies the vitamin or mineral and its most bioavailable form(s).
2. Column 2 states the 1989 recommended daily allowances established by the National Research Council (NRC).
3. Column 3 gives the known toxicity levels.
4. Column 4 summarizes the scientific data on accepted ranges of vitamins and minerals for a daily multivitamin.

VITAMIN AND MINERAL DOSAGE RANGES

Vitamin or Mineral	RDA (1989) Women 25+	Toxicity (RDA 1989)	Range
A (retinol)	4,000 IU	15,000 IU	4,000-15,000 IU
Beta-carotene	—	Unknown	1-15 mg
The 11 most common B vitamins should be taken in a balanced supplement[A]			
Thiamine (B_1)			
25 to 50 years	1.1 mg	Unknown	1.5-200 mg
51+ years	1.0 mg		
Riboflavin (B_2)			
25 to 50 years	1.3 mg	Unknown	1.7-200 mg
51+ years	1.2 mg		
Niacin (B_3) (or niacinamide)			
25 to 50 years	15 mg	3-9 g	20-400 mg
51+ years	13 mg		
B_5 (pantothenic acid)	4-7 mg[B]	10 g	10-300 mg
B_6 (pyridoxine)	1.6 mg	117 mg	2-300 mg
B_{12} (cyanocobalamin)	2 mcg	Unknown	6-300 mcg
Biotin	30-100 mcg[B]	None at 10 mg	25-300 mcg
Choline (lecithin capsules)	—	—	0-100 mg
Folate (folic acid)	180 mcg	None at 10 mg	200 mcg-1 mg
Inositol (lecithin capsules)	—	—	80-300 mg
PABA (para-aminobenzoic acid)	—	—	25-200 mg
C (calcium ascorbate, sodium ascorbate, ascorbic acid	60 mg	Unknown	60-4,000 mg
D (cholecalciferol or D_3)	200 IU	More than 1,000 IU	200-800 IU

Vitamin or Mineral	RDA (1989) Women 25+	Toxicity (RDA 1989)	Range
E (d-alpha tocopherol acetate, or succinate)	8 mg	3,200 mg*	30-800 mg
K (K_1 or K_2)	65 mcg[B]	Unknown	0-100 mcg
Boron	—	—	1.5-3 mg
Calcium[C] (calcium citrate, lactate, gluconate)	800 mg	None at 2,500 mg	200-2,000 mg
Chromium (picolinate or chromic acetate)	50-200 mcg[B]	—	25-200 mcg
Copper (copper gluconate)	1.5-3 mg[B]	None at 5-10 mg	1-3 mg
Fluoride[D]	1.5-4 mg[B] (in diet)	Possibly at 50 mg	—
Iodine (potassium iodide or kelp)	150 mcg	None at 2 mg	25-250 mcg
Iron[E]			
25 to 50 years	15 mg	Unlikely at 75 mg	0-60 mg
51+ years	10 mg		
Magnesium[F] (magnesium gluconate, oxide, or sulfate)	280 mg	Unknown	200-1,000 mg
Manganese (manganese gluconate)	2.0-5.0 mg[B]	None at 8-9 mg	2.5-15 mg
Molybdenum (sodium molybdate)	75-250 mcg[B]	10-15 mg	10-100 mcg

Vitamin or Mineral	RDA (1989) Women 25+	Toxicity (RDA 1989)	Range
Phosphorus[G]	800 mg (in diet)	—	—
Potassium[H]	—	18 g	—
Selenium	55 mcg[B]	1-5 mg	50-200 mcg
Zinc (zinc gluconate or picolinate)	12 mg	120 mg	12-30 mg

NOTE: Postmenopausal women require higher doses of pantothenic acid, niacin, calcium, magnesium, manganese, and vitamin K. Iron doses should be reduced.

*Bendich, A., and Machlin, L. J., "Safety of oral intake of vitamin E," *American Journal of Clinical Nutrition* 48 (1988): 612-19.

[A]The B vitamins must be balanced. High doses of individual vitamins have resulted in symptoms of deficiencies in other B vitamins.

[B]For the ninth edition of the RDAs, the NRC subcommittee created the category "Safe and Adequate Intakes" for nutrients for which there are insufficient data to develop an RDA but for which potentially toxic upper levels are known.

[C]General recommendations for premenopausal women and postmenopausal women on estrogen and hormone replacement therapy are 800 to 1,000 mg per day. The calcium recommendations for postmenopausal women not taking ERT/HRT are 1,000 to 1,500 mg per day. However, the unmistakable trend is toward higher recommendations.

[D]The Food and Nutrition Board recommends that fluoride be added to the public water system if natural levels are less than .7 mg/liter.

[E]Increased ferritin levels and iron levels may cause increased risk of heart disease in postmenopausal women. Certain people are at risk of *hemochromatosis*, a condition that increases iron absorption and results in failure of many organs. (See Chapter 15.)

[F]The generally accepted supplemental ratio of calcium to magnesium is between 2 to 1 and 3 to 1. However, research to the contrary suggests a calcium to magnesium ratio of close to 1 to 2.

[G]The generally accepted calcium to phosphorus ratio is 1 to 1. Lower than a 1 to 2 ratio of calcium to phosphorus can reduce blood calcium levels.

[H]No RDA has been given for potassium, but the minimum requirement is an estimated 1,600 to 2,000 mg. It is probably best to eat an extra serving of fruits or vegetables daily instead of taking a supplement.

WOMAN'S GUIDE™ SUGGESTIONS FOR SUPPLEMENTS

The following suggestions for vitamin and mineral supplements are based on current research. They should be used only as an informational guide for nonpregnant, healthy women over 25. These are not medical recommendations. It is imperative to consult a physician or registered dietitian to determine the proper nutritional supplement for you.

Women Under 40

Vitamin A	5,000 IU	Vitamin K	10 mcg
Beta-carotene	3-5 mg	Boron	3 mg
Thiamine	15 mg	Calcium	1,000-1,500 mg
Riboflavin	15 mg	Chromium	80 mcg
Niacin	30 mg	Copper	2 mg
B_5	25 mg	Fluoride	In water
B_6	50 mg	Iodine	150 mcg
Folic acid	400 mcg	Iron	15 mg
B_{12}	50 mcg	Magnesium	400-600 mg
Biotin	50 mcg	Manganese	5 mg
PABA	30 mg	Molybdenum	15 mcg
Inositol	80 mg	Phosphorus	In diet
Choline	50 mg	Potassium	In diet
Vitamin C	500-1,500 mg	Selenium	50 mcg
Vitamin D	400 IU	Zinc	20 mg
Vitamin E	400-800 mg	Bioflavonoid	100 mg

Women Over 40

Women over 40 and postmenopausal women require larger amounts of the following nutrients:

Niacin	100 mg
Calcium	1,500-2,000 mg
Chromium	100 mcg
Magnesium	500-700 mg
Zinc	30 mg

Iron doses should be reduced to 9 mg. For women taking ERT/HRT calcium recommendation is 1,200 to 1,500 mg.

Woman's Guide™ Nutritional Guidelines

Nutrients

Sodium: 500 mg to no more than 3,000 mg per day.

Fat: Try to consume about 20 percent (certainly less than 30 percent) of total calories, with less than 10 percent from saturated fat; ***reduce hydrogenated fat intake.***

Cholesterol: Less than 250 to 300 mg per day.

Complex carbohydrates: 50 percent to 60 percent of calories.

Fiber: 25 to 30 g per day.

Protein: Less than 15 percent of total calories, or 30 to 70 g. Rely on fish, legumes, and poultry as protein sources rather than on red meat.

Caloric Intake

Women between the ages of 23 and 50 need approximately 2,200 calories per day and should not drop below 1,500 calories. Women over 50 require approximately 1,900 calories per day. These guidelines are approximations; they depend on physical size (petite versus large boned) and activity level (couch potato versus triathlete).

Weight

Maintain desirable weight.

Do not yo-yo diet; lose weight slowly if necessary.

Too thin is 15 percent under average weight for age and height.

Too heavy is 30 percent over average weight for age and height.

Exercise

Three times a week, both aerobic and weight bearing.

Foods to Eat

A wide variety of fresh, unprocessed foods
Soy products
Fish one to two times per week, or an EPA (eicosapentaenoic acid) supplement of 200 to 500 mg per day
Whole grains
Fresh fruits and vegetables
6 to 8 glasses of water per day
Lots of onions and garlic, or take a garlic supplement as directed
Monounsaturated and polyunsaturated oils

Foods to Limit

Alcohol, to no more than one to two drinks per day (if at all)
Sugar to 5 teaspoons per day
Caffeine and chocolate
Saturated oils and fats
Red meats

Things to Try to Avoid

Smoked, salt-cured, and nitrate-cured foods
Processed foods
Hydrogenated oils and fats
Carbonated beverages

Things to Definitely Avoid

Cigarettes
Unnecessary x-rays
Direct sun exposure without protective clothing and sunscreen

Vitamins and Minerals

Select a balanced supplement and take it daily.

Notes

1 Introduction

1. Russell, R. M., and Suter, P. M., "Vitamin requirements of elderly people: An update," *American Journal of Clinical Nutrition* 58 (1993): 4–14.

2 Vitamins and How to Buy Them

1. Wyngaarden, J. B., Smith, L. H., and Bennett, J. C., *Cecil textbook of medicine* (Philadelphia: W. B. Saunders, 1992), 1147.
2. Letter, Penn State Nutritional Center, Benedict House, University Park, PA.
3. Pennington, J. A. T., "Mineral content of foods and total diets: The selected minerals in foods survey, 1982 to 1984," *Journal of the American Dietetic Association* 86 (1986): 876-91.
4. Sempos, C. T., et al., "A two year dietary survey of middle-aged women: Repeated dietary records as a measure of usual intake," *Journal of the American Dietetic Assocation* 84 (1984): 1008–13.
5. Hendler, S. S., *The doctor's vitamin and mineral encyclopedia* (New York: Simon & Schuster, 1990), 431.
6. Ibid.

7. Balch, J. E., and Balch, P. A., *Prescription for nutritional healing* (New York: Avery, 1990), 17; Dunne, L. J., *Nutrition almanac* (New York: McGraw-Hill, 1990), 119-20.
8. Hendler, 430-31.

3 Vitamin A

1. Succari, M., et al., "Influence of sex and age on vitamin A and E status," *Age and Aging* 20 (1991): 413-16.
2. Harman, D., "Free radicals in aging," *Molecular and Cellular Biochemistry* 84 (1988): 155-61.
3. Underwood, B. A., "Vitamin A status and infections," *Nutrition and the M.D.* 17, no. 9 (1991): 1-3.
4. Silverman, A. K., Ellis, C. N., and Voorhees, J. J., "Hypervitaminosis A syndrome: A paradigm of retinoid side effects," *Journal of the American Academy of Dermatology* 16, no. 5 (1987): 1027-39.
5. Menkes, M. S., et al., "Serum beta-carotene, vitamins A and E, selenium, and the risk of lung cancer," *New England Journal of Medicine* 315, no. 20 (1986): 1250-54; Willett, W. C., "Vitamin A and lung cancer," *Nutrition Review* 48 no. 5 (1990): 201-11.
6. Wyngaarden, J. B., Smith, L. H., and Bennett, J. C., *Cecil textbook of medicine* (Philadelphia: W. B. Saunders, 1992), 1178-82.
7. Grahm, S., et al., "Nutritional epidemiology of postmenopausal breast cancer in western New York," *American Journal of Epidemiology* 134, no. 6 (1991): 552-66.
8. Zaridze, D., et al., "Diet, alcohol consumption and reproductive factors in a case-control study of breast cancer in Moscow," *International Journal of Cancer* 48 (1991): 493-501.
9. Lee, H. P., et al., "Risk factors for breast cancer by age and menopausal status: A case-control study in Singapore," *Cancer Causes and Control* 3 (1992): 313-22.
10. Mayne, S. T., Graham, S., and Zheng, T., "Dietary retinol: Prevention or promotion of carcinogenesis in humans?" *Cancer Causes and Control* 2 (1991): 443-50.
11. Hislop, T. G., et al., "Childhood and recent eating patterns and risk of breast cancer," *Cancer Detection and Prevention* 9 (1986): 47-58.
12. Santamaria, L., Dell'Orti, M., and Santamaria, A. B., "Beta-carotene supplementation associated with intermittent retinol administration in the treatment of premenopausal mastodynia," Boll Chim Farmaceutico 128 (1989): 284-87.
13. Mayne et al.; Harris, R. W. C., et al., "A case-control study of dietary carotene in men with lung cancer and in men with other

epithelial cancers," *Nutrition and Cancer* 15 (1991): 63-68; Fontham, E. T. H., "Protective dietary factors and lung cancer," *International Journal of Epidemiology* 19, no. 3 (1990): 32-42; Kalandidi, A., et al., "Passive smoking and diet in the etiology of lung cancer among non-smokers," *Cancer Causes and Control* 1 (1990): 15-21.

14. Willett.
15. Heinonen, O. P., et al., "The effect of beta carotene on the incidence of lung cancer and other cancers in male smokers," *New England Journal of Medicine* 330 (1994): 1029-35.
16. Li, J. Y., et al., "Preliminary report on the results of nutrition prevention trials of cancer and other common diseases among residents in Linxian, China," EBH 15, no. 3 (1993): 165-81.
17. Colditz, G. A., et al., "Increased green and yellow vegetable intake and lowered cancer deaths in an elderly population," *American Journal of Clinical Nutrition* 41 (1985): 32-36.
18. Nowak, R., "Beta-carotene: Helpful or harmful?" *Science* 264 (1994): 500-501.
19. Bosco, D., *The people's guide to vitamins and minerals from A to zinc* (Chicago: Contemporary Books, 1989), 36.
20. Micozzi, M. S., et al., "Plasma carotenoid response to chronic intake of selected foods and beta-carotene supplements in men," *American Journal of Clinical Nutrition* 55 (1992): 1120-25.
21. Perry, S., and O'Hanlan, K., *Natural menopause* (Reading, MA: Addison-Wesley, 1992), 137.
22. Silverman et al.; Wyngaarden et al.
23. Silverman et al.
24. Costas, K., et al., "Use of supplements containing high-dose vitamin A—New York State, 1983-1984," *Journal of the American Medical Association* 257, no. 10 (1987): 1292-97.

4 The B Vitamins

1. Wyngaarden, J. B., Smith, L. H., and Benneett, J. C., *Cecil textbook of medicine* (Philadelphia: W. B. Saunders, 1992), 1171.
2. Ibid., 1172.
3. Luria, M. H., "Effect of low-dose niacin on high-density lipoprotein cholesterol and total cholesterol/high-density lipoprotein cholesterol ratio," *Archives of Internal Medicine* 148 (1988): 2493-95; Carlson, L. A., Hamsten, A., and Asplund, A., "Pronounced lowering of serum levels of lipoprotein Lp(a) in hyperlipidaemic subjects treated with nicotinic acid," *Journal of Internal Medicine* 226 (1989): 271-76.

4. Canner, P. L., et al., "Fifteen year mortality in coronary drug project patients: Long-term benefit with niacin," *Journal of the American College of Cardiology* 8 (1986): 1245–55.
5. McKenney, J. M., et al., "A comparison of the efficacy and toxic effects of sustained- versus immediate-release niacin in hypercholesterolemic patients," *Journal of the American Medical Association* 271, no. 9 (1994): 672–77.
6. Wyngaarten et al., 1175.
7. Coppola, A., Brady, P. G., and Nord, H. J., "Niacin-induced hepatotoxicity: Unusual presentations," *Southern Medical Journal* 87, no. 1 (1994): 30–32.
8. National Research Council, *Recommended dietary allowances* (Washington, D.C.: National Academy Press, 1989), 172.
9. Dalton, K., and Dalton, M. J. T., "Characteristics of pyridoxine overdose neuropathy syndrome," Acta Neurologica Scand 76 (1987): 8–11.
10. Lashner, B. A., Heidenreich, P. A., Su, G. L., Kane, S. V., and Hanauer, S. B., "Effect of folate supplementation on the incidence of dysplasia and cancer in chronic ulcerative colitis," *Gastroenterology* 97 (1989): 255–59.
11. Palca, J., "Agencies split on nutritional advice," *Science* 257 (1992): 1857.
12. Rush, D., "Periconceptional folate and neural tube defect," *American Journal of Clinical Nutrition* 59 (suppl.) (1994): 511s–16s; 511–16.
13. Butterworth, C. E., et al., "Improvement in cervical dysplasia associated with folic acid therapy in users of oral contraceptives," *American Journal of Clinical Nutrition* 35 (1982): 73–82.
14. Potischman, N., "Nutritional epidemiology of cervical neoplasia," *Journal of Nutrition* 123 (1993): 424–29.
15. Joyal, C. C., Lalonde, R., Vikis-Freibergs, V., and Botez, I. M., "Are age-related behavioral disorders improved by folate administration?" *Experimental Aging Research* 19 (1993): 367–76.
16. Sauberlich, H. E., et al., "Folate requirement and metabolism in nonpregnant women," *American Journal of Clinical Nutrition* 46 (1987): 1016–28.
17. Shils, M. E., and Young, V. R., *Modern nutrition in health and disease* (Philadelphia: Lea & Febiger, 1988), 412.
18. Palca.
19. Shojania, A. M., "The effect of oral contraceptives on folate metabolism: III. Plasma clearance and urinary folate excretion," *Journal of Laboratory and Clinical Medicine* 85, no. 2 (1975): 185–90.

20. Milne, D. B., Canfield, W. K., Mahalko, J. R., and Sandstead, H. H., "Effect of oral folic acid supplementations on zinc, copper, and iron absorption and excretion," *American Journal of Clinical Nutrition* 39 (1984): 535-39.
21. Zeisel, S. H., "Choline: An important nutrient in brain development, liver function and carcinogenesis," *Journal of the American College of Nutrition* 11, no. 5 (1992): 473-81.
22. National Research Council, 264.
23. Shils and Young, 447.

5 Vitamin C

1. Bhambhani, M. M., Bates, C. J., and Crisp, A. J., "Plasma ascorbic acid concentrations in osteoporotic outpatients," *British Journal of Rheumatology* 31, no. 2 (1991): 142-43.
2. Dembure, P. P., Janko, A. R., Priest, J. H., and Elsas, L. J., "Ascorbate regulation of collagen biosynthesis in Ehlers-Danlos syndrome, type VI," *Metabolism* 36, no. 7 (1987): 687-91.
3. Thwaites, M., and Dean, S., "Chronic leg ulcers," *Australian Family Physician* 14, no. 4 (1985): 292-98.
4. Williams, R. N., Paterson, C. A., Eakins, K. E., and Bhattacherjee, P., "Ascorbic acid inhibits the activity of polymorphonuclear leukocytes in inflamed ocular tissue," *Experimental Eye Research* 39 (1984): 261-65; Hemila, H., Roberts, P., and Wikstrom, M., "Activated polymorphonuclear leucocytes consume vitamin C," *Federation of European Biochemical Societies Letters* 178, no. 1 (1984): 25-30; Williams, R. N., and Paterson, C. A., "A protective role for ascorbic acid during inflammatory episodes in the eye," *Experimental Eye Research* 42 (1986): 211-18.
5. Frei, B., England, L., and Ames, B. N., "Ascorbate is an outstanding antioxidant in human blood plasma," *Proceedings of the National Academy of Science USA* 86 (1989): 6377-81.
6. Ten-State Nutritional Survey, 1968-1970; National Health and Nutrition Examination Survey—NHANES I, 1971-1974 (studied people age 3-74); NHANES II, 1976-1980 (children 3-11); Hispanic National Health and Nutritional Examination Survey (HNHANES), 1982-1984 (for persons age 4-74). NHANES I and II were designed to supply health and nutritional information for civilian, noninstitutionalized populations of the United States. HNHANES was designed to gather the same information from

three Hispanic populations in Florida, in the Southwest, and in Puerto Rico and New York.

7. Enstrom, J. E., Kanim, L. E., and Klien, M. A., "Vitamin C intake and mortality among a sample of the United States population," *Epidemiology* 3, no. 3 (1992): 194-202.
8. Gey, K. F., Stahelin, H. B., Puska, P., and Evans, A., "Relationship of plasma level of vitamin C to mortality from ischemic heart disease," *Annals of the New York Academy of Science* 488 (1987): 110-23.
9. Erden, F., Gulenc, S., Torun, M., Kocer, Z., Simsek, B., and Nebioglu, S., "Ascorbic acid effect on some lipid fractions in human beings," *Acta Vitaminol Enzymol* 7, no. 1-2 (1985): 131-38.
10. Koumans, A. K. J., and Wildschut, A. J., "Nutrition and atherosclerosis: Some neglected aspects," *Clinical Cardiology* 8 (1985): 547-51.
11. Chen, L. H., Boissonneault, G. A., and Glauert, H. P., "Vitamin C, vitamin E and cancer: Review," *Anticancer Research* 8 (1988): 739-48.
12. Kyrtopoulos, S., "Ascorbic acid and the formation of N-nitroso compounds: Possible role of ascorbic acid in cancer prevention," *American Journal of Clinical Nutrition* 45 (1987): 1344-50.
13. Anderson, R., Theron, A. J., and Ras, G. J., "Ascorbic acid neutralizes reactive oxidants released by hyperactive phagocytes from cigarette smokers," *Lung* 166 (1988): 149-59.
14. Schwartz, J., and Weiss, S. T., "Relationship between dietary vitamin C intake and pulmonary function in the First National Health and Nutrition Examination Survey (NHANES I)," *American Journal of Clinical Nutrition* 59 (1994): 1110-14.
15. Romney, S. L., et al., "Plasma vitamin C and uterine cervical dysplasia," *American Journal of Obstetrics and Gynecology* 151 (1985): 976-80.
16. Pauling, L., "The significance of the evidence about ascorbic acid and the common cold," *Proceedings of the National Academy of Science USA* 68, no. 11 (1971): 2678-81; Hemila, H., "Vitamin C and the common cold," *British Journal of Nutrition* 67 (1992): 3-16; Karlowski, T. R., et al., "Ascorbic acid for the common cold," *Journal of the American Medical Association* 231 (1975): 1038-42.
17. Fulghum, D. D., "Ascorbic acid revisited," *Archives of Dermatology* 113 (1977): 91-92.
18. Bhambhani et al., 142-43.
19. Shils, M. E., and Young, V. R., *Modern nutrition in health and disease* (Philadelphia: Lea & Febiger, 1988), 417-35.

6 VITAMIN D

1. Lukert, B., Higgins, J., and Stoskopf, M., "Menopausal bone loss is partially regulated by dietary intake of vitamin D," *Calcified Tissue International* 51 (1992): 173-79.
2. Lips, P., et al., "The effect of vitamin D supplementation on vitamin D status and parathyroid function in elderly subjects," *Journal of Clinical Endocrinology and Metabolism* 67 (1988): 644-50.
3. Krolner, B., "Seasonal variation of lumbar spine bone mineral content in normal women," *Calcified Tissue International* 35 (1983): 145-47.
4. Krall, E. A., et al., "Effect of vitamin D intake on seasonal variations in parathyroid hormone secretion in postmenopausal women," *New England Journal of Medicine* 321 (1989): 1777-83.
5. Draper, H. H., "Nutrition and osteoporosis," *Canadian Medical Association Journal* 144, no. 7 (1991): 889.
6. Sowers, M. R., Wallace, R. B., and Lemke, J. H., "The association of intakes of vitamin D and calcium with blood pressure among women," *American Journal of Clinical Nutrition* 42 (1985): 135-42.
7. Wyngaarden, J. B., Smith, L. H., and Bennett, J. C., *Cecil textbook of medicine* (Philadelphia: W. B. Saunders, 1992), 1406.

7 VITAMIN E

1. Muller, D. P. R., "Vitamin E: Its role in neurological function," *Postgraduate Medical Journal* 62 (1986): 107-12.
2. Miller, K. L., "Alternatives to estrogen for menopausal symptoms," *Clinical Obstetrics and Gynecology* 35, no. 4 (1992): 884-93.
3. Beard, M., and Curtis, L., *Menopause and the years ahead* (Tucson: Fisher, 1991), 155.
4. (Reading, MA: Addison-Wesley, 1992), 33.
5. (New York: Hearst Books, 1993), 145.
6. Beard and Curtis, 160.
7. Vorherr, H., "Fibrocystic breast disease: Pathophysiology, pathomorphology, clinical picture, and management," *American Journal of Obstetrics and Gynecology* 154, no. 1 (1986): 161-79.
8. Ernster, V. L., et al., "Vitamin E and benign breast 'disease': A double-blind, randomized clinical trial," *Surgery* 97, no. 4 (1985): 490-94; London, R. S., et al., "The effect of vitamin E

on mammary dysplasia: A double-blind study," *Obstetrics and Gynecology* 65, no. 1 (1985): 104-6; Meyer, E. C., et al., "Vitamin E and benign breast disease," *Surgery* 107, no. 5 (1990): 549-51.

9. London, R. S., Murphy, L., and Kitlowski, K. E., "Hypothesis: Breast cancer prevention by supplemental vitamin E," *Journal of the American College of Nutrition* 4 (1985): 559-64.
10. Gerber, M., et al., "Relationship between vitamin E and polyunsaturated fatty acids in breast cancer," *Cancer* 64 (1989): 2347-53.
11. London, R. S., Murphy, L., Kitlowski, K. E., and Reynolds, M. A., "Efficacy of alpha-tocopherol in the treatment of the premenstrual syndrome," *Journal of Reproductive Medicine* 32, no. 6 (1987): 400-404.
12. Bourne, G. H., *Sociological and medical aspects of nutrition* (Basel: Karger, 1988), 170.
13. Li, J. Y., et al., "Preliminary report on the results of nutrition prevention trials of cancer and other common diseases among residents in Linxian, China," EBH 15, no. 3 (1993): 165-81.
14. Menkes, M. S., et al., "Serum beta-carotene, vitamin A and E, selenium, and the risk of lung cancer," *New England Journal of Medicine* 315, no. 20 (1986): 1250-54.
15. Evans, W. J., "Exercise, nutrition and aging," *Journal of Nutrition* 122 (1992): 796-801.
16. Van Der Beek, E. J., "Vitamin supplementation and physical exercise performance," *Journal of Sports Science* 9 (1991): 77-89.
17. Jandak, J., Steiner, M., and Richardson, P. D., "Alpha-tocopherol, an effective inhibitor of platelet adhesion," *Blood* 73, no. 1 (1989): 141-49.
18. Bässler, K. H., "On the problematic nature of vitamin E requirements: Net vitamin E," *Zeitschrift für Ernahrungswissenschaft*, 30 (1991): 174-80.
19. Wyngaarden, J. B., Smith, H. L., and Bennett, J. C., *Cecil textbook of medicine* (Philadelphia: W. B. Saunders, 1992), 1181.
20. Hendler, S. S., *The doctor's vitamin and mineral encyclopedia* (New York: Simon & Schuster, 1990), 108.
21. Bendich, A., and Machlin, L. J., "Safety of oral intake of vitamin $E_{1, 2}$," *American Journal of Clinical Nutrition* 48 (1988): 612-19.
22. Ibid.
23. Wyngaarden et al., 1181.

8 Vitamin K

1. Knapen, M. H. J., Hamulyák, K., and Vermeer, C., "The effect of vitamin K supplementation on circulating osteocalcin (bone Gla protein) and urinary calcium excretion," ***Annals of Internal Medicine*** 111 (1989): 1001-5; Tomita, A., "Postmenopausal osteoporosis Ca study with vitamin K_2," ***Clinical Endocrinology*** 19 (1971): 731-36.
2. Hart, J. P., et al., "Circulating vitamin K_1 levels in fractured neck of femur," ***Lancet*** August 1984, 283; Hodges, S. J., et al., "Depressed levels of circulating menaquinones in patients with osteoporotic fractures of the spine and femur neck," ***Bone*** 12 (1991): 387-89.
3. Hamulyák, K., and Vermeer, C., "Osteocalcin: A vitamin K dependent protein in bone," ***Netherlands Journal of Medicine*** 28 (1985): 305-6; Uchida, K., and Komeno, T., "Relationships between dietary and ingestional vitamin K, clotting factor levels, plasma vitamin K, and urinary Gla.," in ***Vitamin K: Current advances in vitamin K research***, ed. John W. Suttie (New York: Elsevier, 1988), 491.
4. Hodges et al., 387-89.
5. Hendler, S. S., ***The doctor's vitamin and mineral encyclopedia*** (New York: Simon & Schuster, 1990), 109-11.
6. Uchida and Komeno.
7. Shils, M. E., and Young, V. R., ***Modern nutrition in health and disease*** (Philadelphia: Lea & Febiger, 1988), 735; National Research Council, ***Recommended dietary allowances*** (Washington, D.C.: National Academy Press, 1989), 112.

9 Boron

1. Volpe, S. L., Taper, J., and Meacham, S., "The relationship between boron and magnesium status and bone mineral density in the human: A review," ***Magnesium Research*** 6, no. 3 (1993): 291-96; Shils, M. E., and Young, V. R., ***Modern nutrition in health and disease*** (Philadelphia: Lea & Febiger, 1988), 282.
2. Nielsen, F. H., Hunt, C. D., Mullen, L. M., and Hunt, J. R., "Effect of dietary boron on mineral, estrogen, and testosterone in metabolism in postmenopausal women," ***FASEB Journal*** 1 (1987): 394-97.

10 Calcium

1. Amschler, D. H., "Calcium intake: A lifelong proposition," *Journal of School Health* 55, no. 9 (1985): 360-63.
2. Ibid.
3. Mayes, K., *Osteoporosis: Brittle bones and the calcium crisis* (Santa Barbara: Pennant, 1986), 80-81.
4. Heaney, Robert P., "Calcium and vitamin D in human nutrition," in *Calcium, vitamin D, and prevention of colon cancer*, ed. M. Lipkin, H. L. Newmark, and G. Kelloff (Boca Raton: CRC Press, 1991), 9-29.
5. Tesar, R., Notelovitz, M., Shim, E., Kauwell, G., and Brown, J., "Axial and peripheral bone density and nutrient intakes of postmenopausal vegetarian and omnivorous women," *American Journal of Clinical Nutrition* 56 (1992): 699-704; Tylavsky, F. A., and Anderson, J. B., "Dietary factors in bone health of elderly lactoovovegetarians and omnivorous women," *American Journal of Clinical Nutrition* 48 (1988): 842-49; Hunt, I. F., et al., "Bone mineral content in postmenopausal women: Comparison of omnivores and vegetarians," *American Journal of Clinical Nutrition* 50 (1989): 517-23.
6. Ellis, F. R., Holesh, S., and Ellis, J. W., "Incidence of osteoporosis in vegetarian and omnivorous women," *American Journal of Clinical Nutrition* 25 (1972): 555-58; Marsh, A. G., Sanchez, T. V., Michelsen, O., Keiser, J., and Mayor, G., "Cortical bone density of adult lacto-ovovegetarian and omnivorous women," *Journal of the American Dietetic Association* 76 (1980): 148-51.
7. Angus, R. M., Sambrook, P. N., Pocock, N. A., and Eisman, J. A., "Dietary intake and bone density," *Bone and Mineral* 4 (1988): 265-77.
8. Bernstein, D. S., Sadowsky, N., Hegsted, D. M., Guri, C. D., and Stare, F. J., "Prevalence of osteoporosis in high- and low-fluoride areas in North Dakota," *Journal of the American Medical Association* 198, no. 5 (1966): 85-90.
9. Simonen, O., and Laitinen, O., "Does fluoridation of drinking water prevent bone fragility and osteoporosis?" *Lancet*, August 1985, 432-34.
10. Mamelle, N., et al., "Risk-benefit ratio of sodium fluoride treatment in primary vertebral osteoporosis," *Lancet*, August 1988, 361-65.
11. Renner, R. P., Boucher, L. J., and Kaufman, H. W., "Osteoporosis

in postmenopausal women," *Journal of Prosthetic Dentistry* 52, no. 4 (1984): 581-88.

12. Salisbury, J. J., and Mitchell, J. E., "Bone mineral density and anorexia nervosa in women," *American Journal of Psychiatry* 148 (1991): 768-74.
13. Freudenheim, J. L., Johnson, N. E., and Smith, E. L., "Relationships between usual nutrient intake and bone-mineral content of women 35-65 years of age: Longitudinal and cross-sectional analysis," *American Journal of Clinical Nutrition* 44 (1986): 863-76.
14. Holbrook, T. L., and Barrett-Connor, E., "Calcium intake: Covariates and confounders," *American Journal of Clinical Nutrition* 53 (1991): 741-44.
15. Garland, C., Barrett-Connor, E., Rossof, A. H., Shekelle, R. B., Criqui, M. H., and Paul, O., "Dietary vitamin D and calcium and risk of colorectal cancer: A 19 year prospective study in men," *Lancet*, February 1985, 307-25.
16. Sowers, M. R., Wallace, R. B., and Lemke, J. H., "The association of intakes of vitamin D and calcium with blood pressure among women," *American Journal of Clinical Nutrition* 42 (1985): 135-42.
17. Angus et al.; Dawson-Hughes, B., "Calcium supplementation and bone loss: A review of controlled clinical trials," *American Journal of Clinical Nutrition* 54 (1991): 274-80.
18. Reid, I. R., Ames, R. W., Evans, M. C., Gamble, G. D., and Sharpe, S. J., "Effect of calcium supplementation on bone loss in postmenopausal women," *New England Journal of Medicine* 328, no. 7 (1993): 460-64.
19. Prince, R., "The calcium controversy revisited: Implications of new data," *Medical Journal of Australia* 159 (1993): 404-7.
20. Heaney, Robert P., "Calcium and vitamin D in human nutrition," in *Calcium, vitamin D, and prevention of colon cancer*, ed. M. Lipkin, H. L. Newmark, and G. Kelloff (Boca Raton: CRC Press, 1991), 9-29.
21. Wood, R. J., and Serfaty-Lacrosniere, C., "Gastric acidity, atrophic gastritis, and calcium absorption," *Nutrition Reviews* 50, no. 2 (1992): 33-40.
22. National Research Council, *Recommended dietary allowances* (Washington, D.C.: National Academy Press, 1989), 174-184.
23. Dawson-Hughes, B., Seligson, F. H., and Hughes, V. A., "Effects of calcium carbonate and hydroxyapatite on zinc and iron retention in postmenopausal women," *American Clinical Journal* 44, no. 1 (1986): 83-88.

11 Chromium

1. Mertz, W., "Chromium in human nutrition: A review," *Journal of Nutrition* 123 (1993): 626-33.
2. Anderson, R. A., et al., "Effects of supplemental chromium on patients with symptoms of reactive hypoglycemia," *Metabolism* 36, no. 4 (1987): 351-55; Clausen, J., "Chromium induced clinical improvement in symptomatic hypoglycemia," *Biological Trace Element Research* 17 (1988): 229-36.
3. Mossop, R. T., "Trivalent chromium, in atherosclerosis and diabetes," *Central African Journal of Medicine* 37, no. 11 (1991): 369-74.
4. Simonoff, M., "Chromium deficiency and cardiovascular risk," *Cardiovascular Research* 18 (1984): 591-96; Mertz.
5. Mossop; Anderson, R. A., "Chromium metabolism and its role in disease processes in man," *Clinical Physiology and Biochemistry* 4 (1986): 31-41.
6. Mertz, W., personal communication.

12 Copper

1. Hendler, S. S., *The doctor's vitamin and mineral encyclopedia* (New York: Simon & Schuster, 1990), 128.
2. Margalioth, E. J., Schenker, J. G., and Chevion, M., "Copper and zinc levels in normal and malignant tissue," *Cancer* 52 (1983): 868-72.
3. Brandes, J. M., Lightman, A., Drugan, A., Zinder, O., Cohen, A., and Itskovtiz, J., "The diagnostic value of serum copper/zinc ratio in gynecological tumors," *Acta Obstet Gynecol Scand* 62 (1983): 225-29.
4. Kies, C., and Harms, J. M., "Copper absorption as affected by supplemental calcium, magnesium, manganese, selenium and potassium," University of Nebraska Journal Article Series no. 8965, 45-58.
5. National Research Council, *Recommended dietary allowances* (Washington, D.C.: National Academy Press, 1989), 224-30.

13 Fluoride

1. Bernstein, D. S., et al., "Prevalence of osteoporosis in high- and low-fluoride areas in North Dakota," *Journal of the American*

Medical Association 198, no. 5 (1966): 85-90; Simonen, O., and Laitinen, O., "Does fluoridation of drinking water prevent bone fragility and osteoporosis?" *Lancet*, August 1985, 432-33; Mamelle, N., et al., "Risk-benefit ratio of sodium fluoride treatment in primary vertebral osteoporosis," *Lancet*, August 1988, 361-65.
2. Oestreicher, A., "Fluoride's fracture aid disputed," *Medical World News*, October 23, 1989, 42-43.
3. National Research Council, *Recommended dietary allowances* (Washington, D.C.: National Academy Press, 1989), 238.

14 Iodine

1. "Iodine relieves pain of fibrocystic breasts," *Medical World News*, January 11, 1988, 25.
2. Ghent, W. R., Eskin, B. A., Low, D. A., and Hill, L. P., "Iodine replacement in fibrocystic disease of the breast," CJS 36, no. 5 (1993): 453-60.
3. National Research Council, *Recommended dietary allowances* (Washington, D.C.: National Academy Press, 1989), 216.

15 Iron

1. Budoff, P. W., *No more hot flashes* (New York: Warner Books, 1983), 268.
2. Lauffer, R. B., *Iron balance* (New York: St. Martin's, 1991), 27-28.
3. P. 150.
4. Hershko, C., Peto, T. E. A., and Weatherall, D. J., "Iron and infection," *British Medical Journal* 296 (1988): 660-64; Dallman, P. R., "Iron deficiency and the immune response," *American Journal of Clinical Nutrition* 46 (1987): 329-34.

16 Magnesium

1. National Research Council, *Recommended dietary allowances* (Washington, D.C.: National Academy Press, 1989), 188.
2. McLean, R. M., "Magnesium and its therapeutic uses: A review," *American Journal of Medicine* 96 (1994): 63-76.
3. White, J. R., and Campbell, R. K., "Magnesium and diabetes: A

review," *Annals of Pharmacotherapy* 27 (1993): 775-80.
4. Wyngaarden, J. B., Smith, L. H., and Bennett, J. C., *Cecil textbook of medicine* (Philadelphia: W. B. Saunders, 1992), 1138.
5. National Research Council, 189-190.
6. Stanton, M. F., and Lowenstein, F. L., "Serum magnesium in women during pregnancy, while taking contraceptives, and after menopause," *Journal of the American College of Nutrition* 6, no. 4 (1987): 313-19.
7. Schlemmer, A., Podenphant, J., Riis, B. J., and Christiansen, C., "Urinary magnesium in early postmenopausal women," *Magnesium Trace Elements* 92, no. 10 (1991): 34-39.
8. Abraham, G. E., and Grewal, H., "A total dietary program emphasizing magnesium instead of calcium," *Journal of Reproductive Medicine* 35 (1990): 503-7.
9. Sjogren, A., Edvinsson, L., and Fallgren, B., "Magnesium deficiency in coronary artery disease and cardiac arrhythmias," *Journal of Internal Medicine* 226 (1989): 213-22; Dubey, A., and Solomon, R., "Magnesium, myocardial ischaemia and arrhythmias: The role of magnesium in myocardial infarction," *Drugs* 37 (1989): 1-7; Teo, K. K., and Yusuf, S., "Role of magnesium in reducing mortality in acute myocardial infarction," *Drugs* 46, no. 3 (1993): 347-59.
10. Hendler, S. S., *The doctor's vitamin and mineral encyclopedia* (New York: Simon & Schuster, 1990), 158-59.
11. Bosco, D., *The people's guide to vitamins and minerals from A to zinc* (Chicago: Contemporary Books, 1989), 248.

17 Manganese

1. Raloff, J., "Reasons for boning up on manganese," *Science News* 130, no. 13 (1986): 199; Free-Graves, J., et al., "Manganese status of osteoporotics and age-matched, healthy women," *FASEB Journal* 4 (1990), A777.
2. Johnson, P. E., "Manganese and iron metabolism," in *Manganese in health and disease*, ed. D. J. Klimas-Tvantzis (Boca Raton: CRC Press, 1994), 133-43.

18 Molybdenum

1. Sardesai, V. M., "Molybdenum: An essential trace element," *Mayo Clinic Proceedings* 8 (6) (1993): 277-81.

19 Phosphorus

1. National Research Council, *Recommended dietary allowances* (Washington, D.C.: National Academy Press, 1989), 186.
2. Ibid.

20 Potassium

1. Khaw, K., and Barrett-Connor, E., "Dietary potassium and stroke-associated mortality," *New England Journal of Medicine* 316 (1987): 235-40.
2. National Research Council, *Recommended dietary allowances* (Washington, D.C.: National Academy Press, 1989), 256.

21 Selenium

1. Editors of Prevention Magazine, *Understanding vitamins and minerals* (Emmaus, PA: Rodale, 1984), 124-25.
2. Kok, F. J., et al., "Decreased selenium levels in acute myocardial infarction," *Journal of the American Medical Association* 261, no. 8 (1989): 1161-64; Oster, O., et al., "The serum selenium concentration of patients with acute myocardial infarction," *Annals of Clinical Research* 18 (1986): 36-42.
3. Bourne, G. H., *Sociological aspects of nutrition.* (Basel: Karger, 1988), 145-146.
4. Salonen, J. T., et al., "Risk of cancer in relation to serum concentrations of selenium and vitamins A and E: Matched case-control analysis of prospective data," *British Medical Journal* 290 (1985): 417-20.
5. Koskinen, T., Pyykko, K., Kudo, R., Jokela, H., and Punnonen, R., "Serum selenium, vitamin A, vitamin E and cholesterol concentrations in Finnish and Japanese postmenopausal women," *International Journal for Vitamin and Nutrition Research* 57 (1987): 111-14.
6. Salonen et al.
7. National Research Council, *Recommended dietary allowances* (Washington, D.C.: National Academy Press, 1989), 218.
8. Shils, M. E., and Young, V. R., *Modern nutrition in health and disease* (Philadelphia: Lea & Febiger, 1988), 266.
9. National Research Council, 221.

22 Zinc

1. Hendler, S. S., *The doctor's vitamin and mineral encyclopedia* (New York: Simon & Schuster, 1990), 195-96.
2. Milne, D. B., et al., "Ethanol metabolism in postmenopausal women fed a diet marginal in zinc," *American Journal of Clinical Nutrition* 46 (1987): 688-93.
3. Ibid.; McClain, C. J., and Su, L., "Zinc deficiency in the alcoholic: A review," *Clinical and Experimental Research* 7, no. 1 (1983): 5-10.
4. Chilvers, D. C., Jones, M. M., Selby, P. L., Dawson, J. B., and Hodgkinson, A., "Effects of oral ethinyl oestradiol and norethisterone on plasma copper and zinc complexes in postmenopausal women," *Hormone and Metabolic Research* 17 (1985): 532-35.
5. National Research Council, *Recommended dietary allowances* (Washington, D.C.: National Academy Press, 1989), 210-11.

23 Bones

1. Cooper, K. H., *Preventing osteoporosis* (New York: Bantam, 1989), 31-32.
2. Ibid.
3. Brown, S. E., "Osteoporosis: Sorting fact from fallacy," *Network News*, July-August 1988.
4. Christiansen, C., "Prevention and treatment of osteoporosis: A review of current modalities," *Bone* 13 (1992): 35-39; Rubin, C. G., "Southwestern internal medicine conference: Age related osteoporosis," *American Journal of Medical Science* 301, no. 4 (1991): 281-98; Ettinger, B., "A practical guide to preventing osteoporosis," *Western Journal of Medicine* 149 (1988): 691-95.
5. Rubin.
6. Bass, K. M., and Bush, T. L., "Estrogen therapy and cardiovascular risk in women," *Journal* 143 (1991): 33-39.
7. Rubin.
8. Levin, R. M., "The prevention of osteoporosis," *Hospital Practice*, May 15, 1991, 77-97.
9. Wolf, S. M., *Women's health alert* (Reading, MA; Addison-Wesley, 1991), 205.
10. Rubin.
11. Roberts, W. E., et al., "What are the risk factors of osteoporosis?"

National Institute of Dental Research, Grant no. DE09237, 59-62; Renner, R. P., Boucher, L. J., and Kaufman, H. W., "Osteoporosis in postmenopausal women," *Journal of Prosthetic Dentistry* 52, no. 4 (1984): 581-88.

12. Cutler, W. B., and Garcia, C. R., *Menopause: A guide for women and the men who love them* (New York: W. W. Norton 1983), 95.
13. Amschler, D. H., "Calcium intake: A lifelong proposition," *Journal of School Health* 55, no. 9 (1985): 360-63; Gutin, B., and Kasper, M. J., "Can vigorous exercise play a role in osteoporosis prevention?" *Osteoporosis International* 2 (1992): 55-69.
14. Smith, E. L., et al., "Deterring bone loss by exercise intervention in premenopausal and postmenopausal women," *Calcified Tissue International* 44 (1989): 312-21; Grove, K. A., and Londeree, B. R., "Bone density in postmenopausal women: High impact versus low impact exercise," *Medicine and Science in Sports and Exercise*, June 1992, 1190-94.
15. Krall, E. A., and Dawson-Hughes, B., "Walking is related to bone density and rates of bone loss," *American Journal of Medicine* 96 (1994): 20-26.
16. Sinaki, M., Wahner, H. W., Offord, K. P., and Hodgson, S. F., "Efficacy of nonloading exercises in prevention of vertebral bone loss in postmenopausal women: A controlled trial," *Mayo Clinic Proceedings* 64 (1989): 762-69.
17. Levin.
18. Rubin.
19. Marcus, R., et al., "Osteoporosis and exercise in women," *Medicine and Science in Sports and Exercise* 24, no. 6 (1992): 301-7.
20. Sinaki et al.
21. Kanis, J. A., and Passmore, R., "Calcium supplementation of the diet: Not justified by the present evidence," *British Journal of Medicine* 298 (1989): 137-40; Nordin, B. E. C., and Heaney, R. P., "Calcium supplementation of the diet: Justified by present evidence," *British Journal of Medicine* 300 (1990): 1056-62.
22. Toss, G., "Effect of calcium intake versus other life-style factors on bone mass," *Journal of Internal Medicine* 231 (1992): 181-86.
23. Heaney, R. P., and Recker, R. R., "Distribution of calcium absorption in middle-aged women," *American Journal of Clinical Nutrition* 43 (1986): 299-305.
24. Didronel is a registered trademark of Procter & Gamble Pharmaceuticals, Inc., Norwich, New York.

24 Cancer

1. American Cancer Society, *Cancer facts & figures—1992* (Atlanta: American Cancer Society, 1992), 18-20.
2. Ibid., 1-29.
3. "Zeroing in on a breast cancer susceptibility gene," *Science* 259 (1993): 622-23.
4. "Genetic counselling: A preview of what's in store," *Science* 259 (1993): 624.
5. National Alliance of Breast Cancer Organizations, "The diet-breast cancer link," *NABCO News* 2, no. 2 (1988): 1-2.
6. "Focus on breast cancer: Variety of foods being studied as breast cancer preventatives," *Oncology News International*, September 1993, 22-23.
7. National Alliance of Breast Cancer Organizations.
8. Marshall, E., "Search for a killer: Focus shifts from fat to hormones," *Science* 259 (1993): 618-21.
9. National Alliance of Breast Cancer Organizations.
10. Enig, M. G., "Trans fatty acids—an update," *Nutrition Quarterly* 17, no. 4 (1993): 79-95.
11. Marshall.
12. Rovner, S., "Estrogen therapy: Boon or risk factor?" *Washington Post*, August 8, 1989, 8.
13. Marshall; Zeigler, J., "The dilemma of estrogen replacement therapy," *American Health*, April 1992, 68-71.
14. Marshall.
15. Bass, K. M., and Bush, T. L., "Estrogen therapy and cardiovascular risk in women," *Journal of the Louisiana State Medical Society* 143 (1991): 33-39.
16. Henderson, B. E., Ross, R. K., and Pike, M. C., "Hormonal chemoprevention of cancer in women," *Science* 259 (1993): 633-38; Marshall.

25 Estrogen and Hormone Replacement Therapies

1. Testimony of Diane Kennedy before the Fertility and Maternal Drugs Advisory Committee, U.S. Food and Drug Administration, February 1-2, 1990; Wolfe, S., *Women's health alert* (Reading, MA: Addison-Wesley, 1991), 195.
2. Wolfe, 192-222.
3. Grady, D., et al., "Hormone therapy to prevent disease and prolong life in postmenopausal women," *Annals of Internal*

Medicine 117, no. 12 (1992): 1016-37.
4. Lictman, R., "Perimenopausal hormone replacement therapy: Review of the literature," *Journal of Nurse-Midwifery* 36, no. 1 (1991): 30-48.
5. Grady, D., "Women at increased risk for breast cancer," *Annals of Internal Medicine* 117, no. 12 (1992): 1027-37.
6. Rovner, S., "Estrogen therapy: Boon or risk factor?", *Washington Post*, August 8, 1989, Women's Health section.
7. Food and Drug Administration, *How to take your estrogen*, FDA 91-3186 (Washington, D.C.: U.S. Government Printing Office, 1990); *Physicians' desk reference* (Montvale, NJ: Medical Economics Data Production, 1994), 2594.
8. Food and Drug Administration.
9. Notes from K. O'Hanlan, M.D., written in December 1993. Dr. O'Hanlan is an author and physician at Stanford Medical Hospital.
10. Barbach, L., *The pause* (New York: Dutton, 1993), 181-82.
11. Ibid., 105.
12. Perry, S., and O'Hanlan, K. *Natural menopause.* (Reading, MA: Addison-Wesley, 1992), 86-87.
13. Bass, K. M., and Bush, T. L., "Estrogen therapy and cardiovascular risk in women," *Journal* 143 (1991): 33-39.
14. Notes from K. O'Hanlan.
15. Lictman, 30-48.

26 Exercise

1. Wolfe, S. M., *Women's health alert* (Reading, MA: Addison-Wesley, 1991), 211.
2. Evans, W. J., "Exercise, nutrition and aging," *American Institute of Nutrition* 122 (1992): 796-801.
3. American Heart Association, *Exercise and your heart: A guide to physical activity* (Dallas: National Center, 1993), 1-37.
4. Sopko, G., Obarzanek, E., and Stone, E., "Overview of the national heart, lung, and blood institute workshop on physical activity and cardiovascular health," *Medicine and Science in Sports and Exercise* 24, no. 6 (1992): 192-95.
5. American Heart Association, *"Exercise and your heart: A guide to physical activity* (Dallas: National Center, 1993), 1-37. Reproduced with permission. ©1993 American Heart Association.
6. Dubois, E. et al., "Moving for health," in *Ourselves, growing older*, ed. Boston Women's Health Book Collective. (New York:

Simon & Schuster, 1992), 62–75; Perry, S., and O'Hanlan, K., *Natural menopause* (Reading, MA: Addison-Wesley, 1992), 91–93.

7. Kegel, A. M., "Physiologic therapy for urinary stress incontinence," *Journal of the American Medical Association* 146 (1951): 915–17.
8. Perry and O'Hanlan; Dubois et al.
9. Probart, C. K., Bird, P. J., and Parker, K. A., "Diet and athletic performance," *Clinical Nutrition* 77, no. 4 (1993): 757–72.
10. Clarkson, P. M., "Minerals: Exercise performance and supplementation in athletes," *Journal of Sports Science* 9 (1991): 91–116; Haymes, E. M., and Lamanca, J. J., "Iron loss in runners during exercise: Implications and recommendations," *Sports Medicine* 7 (1989): 277–85; Couzy, F., Lafargue, P., and Guezennec, C. Y., "Zinc metabolism in the athlete: Influence of training, nutrition and other factors," *International Journal of Sports Medicine* 11 (1990): 263–66.
11. Kanter, M. M., Nolte, L. A., and Holloszy, J. O., "Effects of an antioxidant vitamin mixture on lipid peroxidation at rest and postexercise," *Journal of Applied Physiology* 74, no. 2 (1993): 965–69; Goldfarb, A. H., "Antioxidants: Role of supplementation to prevent exercise-induced oxidative stress," *Medicine and Science in Sports and Exercise* 25, no. 2 (1993): 232–36.
12. Coyle, E. F., "Timing and method of increased carbohydrate intake to cope with heavy training, competition and recovery," *Journal of Sports Science* 9 (1991): 29–52.
13. Evans, W. J., et al., "Protein metabolism and endurance exercise," *Physician and Sportsmedicine* 11, no. 7 (1983): 63–72; Lemon, P. W. R., "Effect of exercise on protein requirements," *Journal of Sports Science* 9 (1991): 53–70.
14. Position of the American Dietetic Association and the Canadian Dietetic Association: "Nutrition for physical fitness and athletic performance for adults," *Journal of the American Dietetic Association* 93, no. 6 (1993): 691–96.
15. Probart et al.
16. Belko, A. Z., et al., "Effects of exercise on riboflavin requirements of young women," *American Journal of Clinical Nutrition* 37 (1983): 509–17.
17. Van Der Beek, E. J., "Vitamin supplementation and physical exercise performance," *Journal of Sports Science* 9 (1991): 77–89.
18. Ibid.; Simon-Schnass, I., and Pabst, H., "Influence of vitamin E on physical performance," *International Journal of Vitamin and Nutrition Research* 33 (1988): 49–54.

19. Meydani, M., et al., "Protective effect of vitamin E on exercise-induced oxidative damage in young and older adults," *American Journal of Physiology* 33 (1993): R992–R998; Evans et al.
20. Haymes and Lamanca.
21. Probart et al.
22. Couzy et al.
23. Economos, C. D., Bortz, S. S., and Nelson, M. E., "Nutritional practices of elite athletes," *Sports Medicine* 16, no. 6 (1993): 381–99.
24. Probart et al.

27 Fish Oils

1. Sanders, T. A. B., "Fish and coronary artery disease," *British Heart Journal* 57 (1987): 214–19.
2. Fox, P. L., and DiCorleto, P. E., "Fish oils inhibit endothelial cell production of platelet-derived growth factor–like protein," *Science* 241 (1988): 453–56.
3. Dehmer, G. J., et al., "Reduction in the rate of early restenosis after coronary angioplasty by a diet supplemented with n-3 fatty acids," *New England Journal of Medicine* 319, no. 12 (1988): 733–40.
4. Levine, P. H., et al., "Dietary supplementation with omega-3 fatty acids prolongs platelet survival in hyperlipidemic patients with atherosclerosis," *Archives of Internal Medicine* 149 (1989): 1113–16.
5. Knapp, H. R., and FitzGerald, G. A., "The antihypertensive effects of fish oil," *New England Journal of Medicine* 320, no. 16 (1989): 1037–43.
6. Morris, M. C., Sacks, F., and Rosner, B., "Does fish oil lower blood pressure? A meta-analysis of controlled trials," *Circulation* 88 (1993): 523–33.
7. Abbey, M., Clifton, P., Kestin, M., Belling, B., and Nestel, P., "Effect of fish oil on lipoproteins, lecithin: Cholesterol acyltransferase, and lipid transfer protein activity in humans," *Arteriosclerosis* 10 (1990): 85–94.
8. Kromhout, D., Bosschieter, E. B., and Coulander, C., "The inverse relation between fish consumption and 20-year mortality from coronary heart disease," *New England Journal of Medicine* 312, no. 19 (1985): 1205–9.
9. Sanders, T. A. B., "Marine oils: Metabolic effects and role in human nutrition," *Proceedings of the Nutrition Society* 52 (1993): 457–72.

28 Food

1. Stehlin, D., "Women and nutrition: A menu for special needs," *FDA Consumer*, no. 91-2247. (Rockville, MD: Department of Health and Human Services, 1991).
2. U.S. Departments of Agriculture and Health and Human Services, *Dietary guidelines for Americans*, no. 232, 3d ed. (Bethesda, MD: U.S. Departments of Agriculture and Health and Human Services, 1990).
3. American Cancer Society, *Cancer facts and figures—1992* (Atlanta: American Cancer Society, 1992).
4. U.S. Department of Human Services, *Diet, nutrition and cancer prevention: The good news*, no. 87-2878. (Bethesda, MD: U.S. Department of Health and Human Services, National Cancer Institute, 1987).
5. U.S. Departments of Agriculture and Health and Human Services, *Dietary guidelines for Americans*, no. 232, 3d ed. (Bethesda, MD: U.S. Departments of Agriculture and Health and Human Services, 1990).
6. *Cholesterol and your heart: The American Heart Association diet* (Dallas: American Heart Association, 1991).
7. Cutler, B. W., and Garcia, C., *Menopause* (New York: W. W. Norton, 1992), 254.
8. National Research Council, *Recommended dietary allowances* (Washington, D.C.: National Academy Press, 1989), 66; Toss, G., "Effect of calcium intake versus other lifestyle factors on bone mass," *Journal of Internal Medicine* 231 (1992): 181–186.
9. Bobroff, L. B., *Sugar and other sweeteners* (Gainesville: Florida Cooperative Extension Service, University of Florida, 1988), 1-6; Perry, S., and O'Hanlan, K., *Natural menopause* (Reading, MA: Addison-Wesley, 1992), 126–29.
10. Perry and O'Hanlan, 128.
11. Blumenthal, D., *Complex carbohydrates*, FDA no. 90-2230 (Rockville: Department of Health and Human Services, 1989).
12. Bobroff, L. B., *Fiber* (Gainesville: Florida Cooperative Extension Service, University of Florida, 1988).
13. Hallfrisch, J., et al., "Mineral balances of men and women consuming high fiber diets with complex or simple carbohydrates," *Journal of Nutrition* 117 (1987): 48–55.
14. Bobroff, L. B., *Fats* (Gainesville: Florida Cooperative Extension Service, University of Florida, 1988).
15. Enig, M. G., Munn, J., and Keeney, M., "Dietary fat and cancer trends: A critique," *Federation Proceedings* 37 (1978): 2215-22.

16. Ibid.
17. Willett, W. C., "Diet and health: What should we eat?" *Science* 264 (1994): 532-37.
18. Enig, M. G., "Trans fatty acids: An update," *Nutrition Quarterly* 17, no. 4 (1993): 79-95.
19. Willett, W. C., et al., "Intake of *trans* fatty acids and risk of coronary heart disease among women," *Lancet*, March 1993: 581-85; Enig.
20. Enig.
21. School of Public Health, "The new thinking about fats," *University of California Berkeley Wellness Letter*, September 1993.
22. Bobroff, L. B., *Sodium.* (Gainesville: Florida Cooperative Extension Service, University of Florida, 1988), 1-6; American Heart Association, *Salt, sodium and blood pressure: Piecing together the puzzle* (Dallas: National Center, 1979).
23. Stein, P. P., and Black, H. R., "The role of diet in the genesis and treatment of hypertension," *Clinical Nutrition* 77, no. 4 (1993): 831-47.
24. Ibid., 834-36.
25. Mindell, E., *Earl Mindell's vitamin bible* (New York: Warner Books, 1985), 34, 225.
26. Ibid., 145-46; Upton, G. V., "Lipids, cardiovascular disease, and oral contraceptives: A practical perspective," *Fertility and Sterility* 53, no. 1 (1990): 1-12.
27. Perry and O'Hanlan, 144.
28. Somer, E., *Nutrition for women* (New York: Henry Holt, 1993), 232-34.

29 The Female Heart

1. Jaroff, L., "The biggest killer of women: Heart attack," *Time*, November 9, 1992, 72-73; Bass, K. M., and Bush, T. L., "Estrogen therapy and cardiovascular risk in women," *Journal* 143 (1991): 33-39.
2. Utian, W. H., and Jacobowitz, R. S., *Managing your menopause* (New York: Prentice-Hall, 1990), 38-39.
3. Sopko, G., Obarzanek, E., and Stone, E., "Overview of the national heart, lung, and blood institute workshop on physical activity and cardiovascular health," *Medicine and Science in Sports and Exercise* 24, no. 6 (1992): 192-95.
4. Willett, W. C., "Diet and health: What should we eat?" *Science* 264 (1994): 532-37.

30 Herbs

1. Kaldas, R. S., and Hughes, C. L., "Reproductive and general metabolic effects of phytoestrogens in mammals," *Reproductive Toxicology* 3 (1989): 81-89; Murray, M., and Pizzorno, J., *Encyclopedia of Natural Medicine* (Rockland, CA: Prima, 1991), 461-62.
2. Gavaler, J. S., "Alcohol and nutrition in postmenopausal women," *Journal of the American College of Nutrition* 12, no. 4 (1993): 349-56.
3. Fenwick, G. R., and Hanley, A. B., "The genus allium: Part 3," *CRC Critical Reviews in Food Science and Nutrition* 23, no. 1 (1985): 1-73.
4. Fogarty, M., "Garlic's potential role in reducing heart disease," BJCP 47, no. 2 (1993): 64-65.
5. Fenwick and Hanley.
6. Warshafsky, S., Kramer, R. S., and Sivak, S. L., "Effect of garlic on total serum cholesterol: A meta-analysis," *Annals of Internal Medicine* 119 (1993): 599-605.
7. Kiesewetter, H., et al., "Effect of garlic on thrombocyte aggregation, microcirculation, and other risk factors," *International Journal of Clinical Pharmacology Therapy and Toxicology* 29, no. 4 (1991): 151-55.
8. Steinmetz, K. A., et al., "Vegetables, fruit and colon cancer in the Iowa Women's Health Study," *American Journal of Epidemiology* 139, no. 1 (1994): 1-15.
9. Han, J., "Highlights of the cancer chemoprevention studies in China," *Prevention Medicine* 22 (1993): 712-22.
10. Farber, K. S., Barnett, E. D., and Bolduc, G. R., "Antibacterial activity of garlic and onions: A historical perspective," *Pediatric Infectious Disease Journal* 12, no. 7 (1993): 613-14.
11. Elghamry, M. I., and Shihata, I. M., "Biological activity of phytoestrogens," *Veterinary Medicine* (Cairo University, UAR) (1966), 352-57.
12. Murray and Pizzorno.
13. Messina, M., and Barnes, S., "The role of soy products in reducing risk of cancer," *Journal of National Cancer Research* 83, no. 8 (1991): 541-46.
14. Murray and Pizzorno, 461-62.
15. Messina and Barnes.
16. Aldercreutz, H., Honjo, H., Higashi, A., Fotsis, T., Hamalainen, E., Hasegawa, T., and Okada, H., "Urinary excretion of lignans and isoflavonoid phytoestrogens in Japanese men and women consuming a traditional Japanese diet," *American Journal of*

Clinical Nutrition 54 (1991): 1093-1100.
17. Hopkins, M. P., Androff, L., and Benninghoff, A. S., "Ginseng face cream and unexplained vaginal bleeding," *American Journal of Obstetrics and Gynecology* 159, no. 5 (1988): 1121-22.
18. Bennetts, H. W., Underwood, E. J., and Shier, F. L., "A specific breeding problem of sheep on subterranean clover pastures in western Australia," *Australian Veterinary Journal* 22 (1946): 2-12.
19. Setchell, K. D. R, et al., "Dietary estrogens: A probable cause of infertility and liver disease in captive cheetahs," *Gastroenterology* 93 (1987): 225-33.
20. Okwuasaba, F. K., Osunkwo, U. A., Ekwenchi, M. M., Ekpenyong, K. I., Onwukeme, K. E., Olayinka, A. O., Uguru, M. O., and Das, S. C., "Anticonceptive and estrogenic effects of a seed extract of *Ricinus communis* var. *minor*," *Journal of Ethnopharmacology* 34 (1991): 141-45.
21. Vessal, M., Mehrani, H. A., and Omrani, G. H., "Effects of an aqueous extract of Physalis alkekengi fruit on estrus cycle, reproduction and uterine creatine kinase BB-isozyme in rats," *Journal of Ethnopharmacology* 34 (1991): 69-78.
22. Mirkin, G., "Estrogens in yams," *Journal of the American Medical Association* 265, no. 7 (1991): 912.
23. Punnonen, R., and Lukola, A., "Oestrogen-like effect of ginseng," *British Medical Journal* 281 (1980): 281.
24. Albert-Puleo, M., "Fennel and anise as estrogenic agents," *Journal of Ethnopharmacology* 2 (1980): 337-44; Zondek, B., and Bergmann, E., "Phenol methyl ethers as oestrogenic agents," *Biochemstry* 32 (1938): 41-45.

31 Menopause

1. Budoff, P. W., *No more hot flashes* (New York: Warner Books, 1984), 3-9; Perry, S., and O'Hanlan, K., *Natural menopause* (Reading, MA: Addison-Wesley, 1992), 17.
2. Perry and O'Hanlan, 9.
3. Utian, W. H., and Jacobowitz, R. S., *Managing your menopause* (New York: Prentice-Hall, 1990), 35.
4. Perry and O'Hanlan, 90.
5. Sheehy, G., *Silent passages* (New York: Random House, 1992), 23.
6. Perry and O'Hanlan, 28-35.
7. Weber, G., "A season for sex," *Healthsharing*, Fall-Winter 1990, 18-21; Perry and O'Hanlan, 84-87.
8. Perry and O'Hanlan, 32.

32 Premenstrual Syndrome (PMS)

1. Martorano, J., Morgan, M., and Fryer, W., *Unmasking PMS: The complete medical treatment plan* (New York: M. Evans, 1993), 201.
2. Abraham, G. E., "Nutritional factors in the etiology of the premenstrual tension syndromes," *Journal of Reproductive Medicine* 28, no. 7 (1983): 446-64.
3. Abraham, G. E., and Hargrove, J. T., "Effect of vitamin B-6 on premenstrual symptomatology in women with premenstrual tension syndromes: A double blind crossover study," *Infertility* 3, no. 2 (1980): 155-65.
4. Dalton, K., and Dalton, M. J. T., "Characteristics of pyridoxine overdose neuropathy syndrome." *Acta Neurol Scand*, 76 (1987): 8-11.
5. Dalton, K., *The premenstrual syndrome and progesterone therapy* (Chicago: Yearbook Medical Publishers, 1984), 124; Martorano et al., 172.
6. Abraham, 446-64.
7. Martorano et al., 171.
8. Mindell, E., *Earl Mindell's vitamin bible* (New York: Warner Books, 1985), 235.
9. Maxson, W. S., and Hargrove, J. T., "Bioavailability of oral micronized progesterone," *Fertility and Sterility* 44, no. 5 (1985): 622-26; Martorano, J. T., Ahlgrimm, M., and Myers, D., "Differentiating between natural progesterogens: Clinical implications for premenstrual syndrome management," *Comprehensive Therapy* 19, no. 3 (1993): 96-98.
10. Dennerstein, L., et al., "Progesterone and the premenstrual syndrome: A double blind crossover trial," *British Medical Journal* 290 (1985): 1617-21.
11. Martorano et al, 194.
12. Moline, M. L., "Pharmacologic strategies for managing premenstrual syndrome," *Clinical Pharmacology* 12 (1993): 181-96.
13. Plouffe, L., et al., "Premenstrual syndrome update on diagnosis and management," *Female Patient* 19 (1994): 53-58.

33 Skin and Aging

1. Novick, N. L., *Super skin* (New York: Clarkson N. Potter, 1988), 4.
2. Wyngaarden, J. B., Smith, L. H., and Bennett, J. C., *Cecil textbook of medicine* (Philadelphia: W. B. Saunders, 1992), 2282-86.
3. Kurban, R. S., and Bhawan, J., "Histologic changes in skin associated with aging," *Journal of Dermatologic Surgery and Oncology* 16 (1990): 909.

4. Ibid., 908–14.
5. Ibid., 911.
6. Ibid.
7. Lavker, R. M., Zheng, P., and Dong, G., "Morphology of aged skin," *Dermatologic Clinics* 4, no. 3 (1986): 379–89.
8. Downing, D. T., Stewart, M. E., and Strauss, J. S., "Changes in sebum secretion and the sebaceous gland," *Dermatologic Clinics* 4, no. 3 (1986): 419–23.
9. Warren, R., et al., "Age, sunlight, and facial skin: A histologic and quantitative study," *Journal of the American Academy of Dermatology* 25 (1991): 751–60.
10. Lavker et al.
11. Sams, W. M., "Sun-induced aging: Clinical and laboratory observations in man," *Dermatologic Clinics* 4, no. 3 (1986): 509–16.
12. Lavker et al.
13. Pathak, M. A., "Ultraviolet radiation and the development of non-melanoma and melanoma skin cancer: Clinical and experimental evidence," *Skin Pharmacology* 4, no. 1 (1991): 85–94.
14. American Cancer Society, *Cancer facts and figures—1992* (Atlanta: American Cancer Society, 1992), 17–20.
15. Ibid.
16. Perry, S., and O'Hanlan, K., *Natural menopause* (Reading, MA: Addison-Wesley, 1992), 169–70.
17. Burke, K. E., "Facial wrinkles: Prevention and nonsurgical correction," *Postgraduate Medicine* 88, no. 1 (1990): 207–28.
18. Registered trademark of Ortho Pharmaceutical Corporation.
19. Registered trade name of Berner Ltd., Finland.
20. Registered trade name of Scandinavian Natural Health and Beauty Products, Inc.
21. Eskelinen, A., and Santalhti, J., "Special natural cartilage polysaccharides for the treatment of sun-damaged skin in females," *Journal of International Medical Research* 20 (1992): 99–105.
22. Pinski, K. S., and Roenigk, H. H., "Autologous fat transplantation," *Journal of Dermatologic Surgery and Oncology* 18 (1992): 179–184.
23. Novick, 209–10; Zaias, N., *The nail in health and disease* (Norwalk, CT: Appleton & Lange, 1990), 11, 164.
24. Ibid., 165.
25. Hendler, S. S., *The doctor's vitamin and mineral encyclopedia* (New York: Simon & Schuster, 1990), 277–78; Klein, A. D., and Penneys, N. S., "Aloe vera," *Journal of the American Academy of Dermatology* 18 (1989): 714–20.
26. Olsen, E. A., et al., "Tretinoin emollient cream: A new therapy for photodamaged skin," *Journal of the American Academy of*

Dermatology 26 (1992): 215–24; Brodell, L. P., Asselin, D., and Brodell, R. T., "Reversible ectropion after long-term use of topical tretinoin on photodamaged skin," *Journal of the American Academy of Dermatology* 27, no. 4 (1992): 621–22.

34 Weight

1. Jacobowitz, R. S., *150 most-asked questions about menopause* (New York: Hearst Books, 1993), 200.
2. Perry, S., and O'Hanlan, K., *Natural menopause* (Reading, MA: Addison-Wesley, 1992), 122.
3. Lapidus, L., et al., "Dietary habits in relation to incidence of cardiovascular disease and death in women: A 12-year follow-up of participants in the population study of women in Gothenburg, Sweden," *Journal of Clinical Nutrition* 44 (1986): 444–48.
4. American Heart Association, *Heart and stroke facts* (Dallas: National Center, 1992), 38.
5. Hocman, G., "Prevention of cancer: Restriction of nutritional energy intake (joules)," *Comparative Biochemistry and Physiology* 91, no. 2 (Autumn 1988): 209–220; American Cancer Association, *Cancer figures and facts—1992* (Atlanta: National Center), 20.
6. Tsukamoto, H., and Sano, F., "Body weight and longevity: Insurance experience in Japan," *Diabetes Research and Clinical Practice* 10 (1990): 119–25.
7. Rissanen, A., et al., "Weight and mortality in Finnish women," *Journal of Clinical Epidemiology* 44, no. 8 (1991): 787–95.
8. Morley, J. E., "Nutritional problems of the elderly," Biol Asoc Medical Clinic Puerto Rico 79, no. 12 (1987): 505–7.
9. Goldstein, D. J., "Beneficial health effects of modest weight loss," *International Journal of Obesity* 16 (1992): 397–415.
10. Lee, I., and Paffenbarger, R. S., "Change in body weight and longevity," *Journal of the American Medical Association* 268 (1992): 2045–49.
11. Levy, A. S., and Heaton, A. W., "Weight control practices of U.S. adults trying to lose weight," *Annals of Internal Medicine* 119 (1993): 661–66.
12. Utian, W. H., and Jacobowitz, R. S., *Managing your menopause* (New York: Prentice-Hall, 1990), 101–2.
13. "Theories on yo-yo dieting unwind," *Tufts University Diet & Nutrition Newsletter* 12, no. 10, December 1994.
14. American Diabetes Association and American Dietetic Association. *Nutrition guide for professionals: Diabetes education and meal planning* (1988), 29.

BIBLIOGRAPHY

Abdeljaber, M. H., et al. "The impact of vitamin A supplementation on morbidity: A randomized community trial." *American Journal of Public Health* 81, no. 12 (1991): 1654–56.

Ackerman, A. B. *Histologic diagnosis of inflammatory skin diseases.* Philadelphia: Lea & Febiger, 1978.

Ahroni, A., et al. "Hair chromium content of women with gestational diabetes compared with nondiabetic pregnant women." *American Journal of Clinical Nutrition* 55 (1992): 104-7.

American Heart Association. *Heart and stroke facts.* Dallas: National Center, 1992.

Balch, J. F., and Balch, P. A. *A prescription for nutritional healing.* New York: Avery, 1990.

Balfour, J. A., and Heel, R. C. "Transdermal estradiol: A review of its pharmacodynamic and pharmacokinetic properties, and therapeutic efficacy in the treatment of menopausal complaints." *Drugs* 40, no. 4 (1990): 561-82.

Barbach, L. *The pause.* New York: Dutton, 1993.

Bates, C. J., et al. "The discrepancy between normal folate intakes and the folate RDA." *Human Nutrition; Applied Nutrition* 36 (Autumn 1982): 422-29.

Beard, M., and Curtis, L. *Menopause and the years ahead.* Tucson: Fisher, 1991.

Bishop, N., Schorah, C. J., and Wales, J. K. "The effect of vitamin C supplementation on diabetic hyperlipidaemia: A double-blind, crossover study." *Diabetic Medicine* 2 (1985): 121-24.

Bonjour, J. P., "Biotin in human nutrition." *Annals of the New York Academy of Science* 447 (1985): 97-104.

Bordia, A., and Verma, S. K. "Effect of vitamin C on platelet adhesiveness and platelet aggregation in coronary artery disease in patients." *Clinical Cardiology* 8 (1985): 552-54.

Bosco, D. *The people's guide to vitamins and minerals from A to zinc.* Chicago: Contemporary Books, 1989.

Boston Women's Health Book Collective. *Ourselves, growing older.* New York: Simon & Schuster, 1992.

Bourne, G. H. *Sociological and medical aspects of nutrition.* Basel: Karger, 1988.

Brandes, J. M., et al. "The diagnostic value of serum copper/zinc ratio in genealogical tumors." Acta Obstetrics Gynecologics Scandinavia, 62 (1983): 225-29.

Bricklan, M. *Natural healing.* Emmaus, PA: Rodale, 1983.

Budoff, P. W. *No more hot flashes.* New York: Warner Books, 1984.

Burroughs, C. D., Bern, H. A., and Stokstad, E. L. R. "Prolonged vaginal cornification and other changes in mice treated neonatally with coumestrol, a plant estrogen." *Journal of Toxicology and Environmental Health* 15 (1985): 51-61.

Chilvers, D. C., Jones, M. M., Selby, P. L., Dawson, J. B., and Hodgkinson, A. "Effects of oral ethinyl oestradiol and norethisterone on plasma copper and zinc complexes in postmenopausal women. *Hormone and Metabolic Research* 17 (1985): 532-35.

Clark, L. C. "The epidemiology of selenium and cancer." *Federation Proceedings* 44, no. 9 (1985): 2584-89.

Clement, I. P. "Selenium inhibition of chemical carcinogenesis." *Federation Proceedings* 44, no. 9 (1985): 2573-78.

Clement, I. P. "Interaction of vitamin C and selenium supplementation in the modification of mammary carcinogenesis in rats." JNCL, 77 (1986): 299-303.

Cooper, J. A., et al. "Risk factors for breast cancer by oestrogen receptor status: A population-based case-control study." *Cancer* 39 (1989): 119-25.

Costello, C. H., and Lynn, E. V. "Estrogenic substances from plants: I. Glycyrrhiza." *Journal of the American Pharmaceutical Association* (1949): 177-80.

Crawford, T., et al. "Prevalence and pathological changes of ischemic heart-disease in a hard-water and in a soft-water area." *Lancet*, February 1967, 229-32.

Cutler, W. B., and Garcia, C. *Menopause: A guide for women and the men who love them.* New York: W. W. Norton, 1992.

Czeizel, A. E., and Dudas, I. "Prevention of the first occurence of neural-tube defects by periconceptional vitamin supplementation." *New England Journal of Medicine* 327 (1992): 1832-5.

Dalton, K. *The premenstrual syndrome and progesterone therapy.* Chicago: Yearbook Medical Publishers, 1984.

de Souza, M. "The colors of menopause." *Healthsharing*, Winter 1990, 14-17.

Dhur, A., Galan, P., and Hercberg, S. "Iron status: Immune capacity and resistance to infections." *Comparative Biochemistry and Physiology* 94, no. 1 (1989): 11-19.

Dodds, E. C., and Lawson, W. "A simple aromatic estrogenic agent with an activity of the same order as estrogen." *Nature* 137 (1936): 627-28.

Duncan, L. *Coming to terms with PMS.* Riviera Beach, FL: Rosecott, 1986.

Eagan, A. B. "The estrogen fix." *Ms.*, April 1989, 38-41.

Editors of Prevention Magazine. *Healing remedies and techniques.* Emmaus, PA: Rodale, 1992.

Elmougy, S. A., Hassanein, R. R., and Elghamry, M. I. "Biological activity of phytoestrogens." *Veterinary Medicine* 19 (1972): 337-42.

El-Yazigi, A., Hannan, N., and Raines, D. A. "Urinary excretion of chromium, copper, and manganese in diabetes mellitus and associated disorders." *Diabetes Research* 18 (1991): 129-34.

"The estrogen question." *Consumer Report*, September 1991.

Favennec, L. "The biological effects of retinoids on cell differentiation and proliferation." *Journal of Clinical Chemistry and Clinical Biochemistry* 26, no. 8 (1988): 479-89.

FDA Consumer. *Some facts and myths about vitamins.* No 79-2117. Washington, D.C.: U.S. Department of Health and Human Services, 1979.

Foulke, J. E. "Cosmetic ingredients: Understanding the puffery." *FDA Consumer*, May 1992, 1-4.

Gey, K. F. "On the antioxidant hypothesis with regard to arteriosclerosis." *Bibltheca Nutrition Dietary* 37 (1986): 53-91.

Gey, K. F., Brubacher, G. B., and Stahelin, H. B. "Plasma levels of antioxidant vitamins in relation to ischemic heart disease and cancer." *American Journal of Clinical Nutrition* 45 (1987): 1368-77.

Gillespie, C. *Hormones, hot flashes and mood swings.* New York: Harper Perennial, 1989.

Gladstar, R. *Herbal healing for women.* New York: Simon & Schuster, 1993.

Grahm, S., et al. "Diet in the epidemiology of breast cancer." *American Journal of Epidemiology* 116, no. 1 (1982): 68-75.

Gray, H., and Hoss, C. M. *Anatomy of the human body*. Philadelphia: Lea & Febiger, 1970.

Greenwood, S. *Menopause naturally*. Volcano, HI: Volcano, 1989.

Griffith, H. W. *Complete guide to prescription and nonprescription drugs*. Los Angeles: Body Press, 1988.

Hausman, P. *The calcium bible: How to have better bones your whole life*. New York: Rawson, 1985.

Heaney, R. P. *Calcium and common science*. New York: Doubleday, 1988.

Heidrich, F., and Thompson, R. S. "Osteoporosis prevention: Strategies applicable for general population groups." *Journal of Family Practice* 25, no. 1 (1987): 33-39.

Hemila, H. "Vitamin C and plasma cholesterol." *Critical Review of Food* Sci Nutr, 32, no. 1 (1992): 33-57.

Hendler, S. S. *The doctor's vitamin and mineral encyclopedia*. New York: Simon & Schuster, 1990.

Hislop, T. G., et al. "Influence of estrogen receptor status on dietary risk factors for breast cancer." *Canadian Medical Assocation Journal* 138 (1988): 424-30.

Holt, L. H., and Weber, M. *WomenCare*. New York: Random House, 1982.

Honoré, L. H., Salkie, M. L., and Jajckay, F. L. "The influence of anatomical site and hormonal status on the copper and zinc levels of human uterine smooth muscle." *Clinical Biochemistry* 19 (1986) 46-48.

Hunter, D. J., et al. "A prospective study of consumption of vitamins A, C, and E and breast cancer risk." *SER Abstracts*, Harvard University, 715.

"An interpretive review of recent nutrition research." *Dairy Council Digest* 61, no. 5 (1990): 25-30.

Jacobowitz, R. S. *150 most-asked questions about menopause*. New York: Hearst Books, 1993.

Jamison, J. R. "Counteracting nutritional misinformation: A curricular proposal." *Journal of Manipulative Physiological Therapeutics* 13, no. 8 (1990): 454-61.

Kamidao, H., Matsuzawa, Y., and Tarui, S. "Lipid composition of platelets from patients with atherosclerosis: Effect of purified eicosapentaenoic acid ethyl ester administration." *Lipids* 23 (1988): 917-23.

Kappus, H., and Diplock, A. T. "Tolerance and safety of vitamin E: A toxicological position report." *Free Radical Biology and Medicine* 13 (1992): 55-74.

Kitts, D. D. "Studies on the estrogenic activity of a coffee extract." *Journal of Toxicology and Environmental Health* 20 (1987): 37-49.

Kok, F. J., et al. "Selenium status and chronic disease mortality: Dutch epidemiological findings." *International Journal of Epidemiology* 16, no. 2 (1987): 329-31.

Kok, F. J. "Serum selenium, vitamin antioxidants, and cardiovascular mortality: A 9-year follow-up study in the Netherlands." *American Journal of Clinical Nutrition* 45 (1987): 463-68.

Levin, R. M. "The prevention of osteoporosis." *Hospital Practice*, May 1991, 77-97.

Lewis, J. S., et al. "Effect of long-term ingestion of polyunsaturated fat, age, plasma cholesterol, diabetes mellitus, and supplemental tocopherol upon plasma tocopherol." *American Journal of Clinical Nutrition* 26 (1973): 136-43.

Lian, J. B. "Osteocalcin: Functional studies and postulated role in bone resorption." In *Vitamin K: Current advances in vitamin K research*. Ed. J. W. Suttie. New York: Elsevier, 1988.

Lieberman, S., and Bruning, N. *The real vitamin and mineral book*. New York: Avery, 1990.

Lundh, T. J. O., Petterson, H. I., and Martinsson, K. A. "Comparative levels of free and conjugated plant estrogens in blood plasma of sheep and cattle fed estrogenic silage." *Journal of Agricultural Food Chemistry* 38 (1990): 1530-34.

Margalioth, E. J., Schenker, J. G., and Chevion, M. "Copper and zinc levels in normal and malignant tissues." *Cancer* 52 (1983): 868-72.

Marshall, M. W. "The nutritional importance of biotin: An update." *Nutrition Today*, November-December 1987, 26-30.

McLaren, D. S. "Vitamin A supplementation and mortality." *Lancet* 338 (1991): 1208-9.

McLennan, S., et al. "Deficiency of ascorbic acid in experimental diabetes." *Diabetes* 37 (1988): 359-61.

Miksicek, R. J. "Commonly occurring plant flavonoids have estrogenic activity." *Molecular Pharmacology* 44 (1993): 37-43.

Mindell, E. *Earl Mindell's vitamin bible*. New York: Warner Books, 1985.

Moline, M. L. "Pharmacologic strategies for managing premenstrual syndrome. *Clinical Pharmacology* 12 (1993): 181-96.

Monsen, E. R., et al. "Estimation of available dietary iron." *American Journal of Clinical Nutrition* 31 (1978): 134-41.

Mori, T. A., et al. "New findings in the fatty acid composition of individual platelet phospholipids in man after dietary fish oil supplementation." *Lipids* 22 (1987): 744-50.

Munro, H. N. "Evolving scientific bases for the recommended dietary allowances: A critical look at methodologies." *American Journal of Clinical Nutrition* 41 (1985): 148-54.

National Research Council. *Recommended daily allowances*. Washington, D.C.: National Academy Press, 1989.

National Women's Health Network. "Alternatives to hormone use." *A Friend Indeed* 5, no. 5 (1988): 1-10.

Nielsen, F. H. "Boron: An overlooked element of potential nutritional importance." *Nutrition Today*, January-February 1988, 394-97.

Olson, J. A. "Carotenoids, vitamin A and cancer." *Journal of Nutrition* 116 (1986): 1127-30.

"Over-the-counter niacin." Editorial. *Journal of the American Medical Association* 271, no. 9 (1994): 709-10.

Pauling, L. "The significance of the evidence about ascorbic acid and the common cold." *Proceedings of the National Academy of Science* 68, no. 11 (1971): 2678-81.

Peck, W. A., and Avioli, L. V. *Osteoporosis: The silent thief.* Washington, D.C.: AARP Books, 1988.

Perry, S., and O'Hanlan, K. *Natural menopause.* Reading, MA: Addison-Wesley, 1992.

Pilch, S. M. "Analysis of vitamin A data from the health and nutrition examination surveys." *Journal of Nutrition* 117 (1987): 636-40.

Randal, J. E. "Deciding on hormone therapy." *Newsday*, August 1989.

Redei, E., and Freeman, E. W. "Preliminary evidence for plasma adrenocorticotropin levels as biological correlates of premenstrual symptoms." *Acta Endocrinologica* 128 (1993): 536-42.

Reginster, J. Y., et al. "Preliminary report of increased serum magnesium in postmenopausal osteoporosis." *Magnesium* 8 (1989): 106-9.

Reitz, R. *Menopause: A positive approach.* Raduor, PA: Chilton, 1977.

Richardson, S., Gerber, M., and Cenee, S. "The role of fat, animal protein and some vitamin consumption in breast cancer: A case control study in southern France." *International Journal of Cancer* 48 (1991): 1-9.

Robbins, S. L. *Pathologic basis of disease.* Philadelphia: W. B. Saunders, 1974.

Rook, A., Wilkinson, D. S., and Ebling, F. J. G. *Textbook of dermatology.* Oxford: Blackwell Scientific Publications, 1979.

Salonen, J. T., et al. "Association between serum selenium and the risk of cancer." *American Journal of Epidemiology* 120, no. 3 (1984): 342-49.

Salonen, J. T., et al. "Risk of cancer in relation to serum concentrations of selenium and vitamins A and E: Matched case-control analysis of prospective data." *British Medical Journal* 290 (1985): 417-20.

Sarbaddhukari, S. N. "Hypervitaminoses." *Journal of Indian Medical Association* 91, no. 7 (1993): 1951.

Schaumburg, H., et al. "Sensory neuropathy from pyridoxine abuse." *New England Journal of Medicine* 309, no. 8 (1983): 445-48.

Seigal, D., et al. "Menopause: Entering our third age." *Ourselves, growing older*, ed. Boston Women's Health Book Collective. New York: Simon & Schuster, 1992.

Setchell, K. D. R., Welsh, M. B., and Lim, C. K. "High performance liquid chromatographic analysis of phytoestrogens in soy protein preparations with ultraviolet, electrochemical and thermospray mass spectrometric detection." *Journal of Chromatography* 386 (1987): 315-23.

Sheehy, Gail. *Silent passages*. New York: Random House, 1992.

Shils, M. E., and Young, V. R. *Modern nutrition in health and disease*. Philadelphia: Lea & Febiger, 1988.

Simard, A., Vobecky, J., and Vobecky, J. S. "Vitamin D deficiency and cancer of the breast: An unprovocative ecological hypothesis." *Canadian Journal of Public Health* 82 (1991): 300-303.

Singh, R. B. "Dietary strategies for risk-factor modification to prevent cardiovascular diseases." *Nutrition* 7, no. 3 (1991): 210-14.

Sitruk-Ware, R., et al. "Oral micronized progesterone." *Contraception* 36, no. 4 (1987): 373-401.

Sowers, M. R., and Wallace, R. B. "Retinol, supplemental vitamin A and bone status." *Journal of Clinical Epidemiology* 43, no. 7 (1990): 693-99.

Spencer, H., Norris, C., and Osis, D. "Further studies of the effect of zinc on intestinal absorption of calcium in man," *Journal of the American College of Nutrition* 11, no. 5 (1992): 561-66.

Spodnik, J. P. *The 35 good health guide: The prime of life program for women over 35*. New York: Harper & Row, 1989.

Stauber, P. M. "A longitudinal study of the relationship between vitamin A supplementation and plasma retinol, retinyl esters, and liver enzyme activities in a healthy elderly population." *American Journal of Clinical Nutrition* 54 (1991): 873-83.

Thompson, D. S. *Everyone's health*, 73. New York: Prentice-Hall, 1980.

Thompson, D. S. *Everywoman's health: a complete guide to body and mind*. New York: Prentice-Hall, 1985.

Tierra, L. *The way of herbs*. New York: Pocket Books, 1980.

Utian, W. H., and Jacobowitz, R. *Managing your menopause*. New York: Fireside, 1990.

Vandewoode, M. F. J., and Vandewoode, M. G. "Vitamin E status in a normal population: The influence of age." *Journal of the American College of Nutrition* 6, no. 4 (1987): 307-11.

von Kries, R. "Vitamin K prophylaxis: A useful public health measure?" *Paediatric and Perinatal Epidemiology* 6 (1992): 7-13.

Vyas, D., and Chandra, R. K. "Vitamin A and immunocompetence." Newfoundland: Janeway Child Health Center.

Wald, N. J. and Bower, C. "Folic acid, pernicious anaemia, and prevention of neural tube defects." *Lancet* 343 (1994): 307.

Weber, G. "A season for sex." *Healthsharing*, Fall-Winter 1990, 18-21.

Willett, W. C., et al. "Dietary fat and fiber in relation to risk of breast cancer." *Journal of the American Medical Association* 268, no. 15 (1992): 2037-44.

Wood, R. J., and Zheng, J. J., "Milk consumption and zinc retention in postmenopausal women," *Journal of Nutrition* 120 (1990): 389-403.

Wyngaarden, J. B., Smith, L. H., and Bennett, J. C. *Cecil textbook of medicine*. Philadephia: W. B. Saunders, 1992.

Ziegler, J. "The dilemma of estrogen replacement therapy." *American Health*, April 1992, 68-71.

INDEX

Italic page numbers indicate pages on which definitions of terms appear.